most currented.
11/11/2021
GRL

Clinical Guide

to the Treatment
of the Mentally Ill
Homeless Person

D1568266

Clinical Guide to the Treatment of the Mentally Ill Homeless Person

Edited by

Paulette Marie Gillig, M.D.

Professor, Boonshoft School of Medicine,
Department of Psychiatry, Wright State University, Dayton, Ohio

Hunter L. McQuistion, M.D.

Adjunct Associate Clinical Professor, Department of Psychiatry,
The Mount Sinai School of Medicine, New York, New York

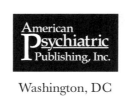

Washington, DC
London, England

To purchase 25–99 copies of this or any other APPI title at a 20% discount, please contact APPI Customer Service at appi@psych .org or 800-368-5777. For 100 or more copies of the same title, please e-mail us at bulksales@psych.org for a price quote.

Copyright © 2006 American Psychiatric Publishing, Inc.
ALL RIGHTS RESERVED

Manufactured in the United States of America on acid-free paper
10   09   08   07   06   5   4   3   2   1
First Edition

Typeset in Adobe's Christiana and Baskerville.

American Psychiatric Publishing, Inc.
1000 Wilson Boulevard
Arlington, VA 22209-3901
www.appi.org

Library of Congress Cataloging-in-Publication Data

Clinical guide to the treatment of the mentally ill homeless person /
    edited by Paulette Marie Gillig, Hunter L. McQuistion. —1st ed.
       p. ; cm.
    Includes bibliographical references and index.
    ISBN 1-58562-251-6 (pbk. : alk. paper)
       1. Homeless persons—Mental health. 2. Homeless persons—Psychology.
    3. Homeless persons—Mental health services. 4. Community mental health
    services. I. Gillig, Paulette Marie, 1949– . II. McQuistion, Hunter L., 1952– .
       [DNLM: 1. Community Mental Health Services—methods. 2. Mentally Ill
    Persons—psychology. 3. Homeless Persons—psychology. 4. Mental Disorders—
    therapy.   WM 30 C6407 2006]
    RC451.4.H64C555 2006
    362.2086'942—dc22

                                                        2006014398

British Library Cataloguing in Publication Data
A CIP record is available from the British Library.

Dr. Gillig dedicates this book to the memory of her mother, Marie.
Dr. McQuistion dedicates this work to Judy: without whom
homelessness would have had new meaning.

CONTENTS

CONTRIBUTORS

Paulette Marie Gillig, M.D., Ph.D. (editor)

Professor of Psychiatry and Community Psychiatry, Boonshoft School of Medicine, Wright State University, Dayton, Ohio; Director of the Division of Rural Psychiatry, Wright State University. Dr. Gillig is also Consulting Psychiatrist to Consolidated Care, Inc., West Liberty, Ohio. Consolidated Care provides comprehensive mental health, drug, and alcohol services to adults and children, homeless and domiciled, in several rural counties in Ohio. Twelve years ago, Consolidated Care, Inc., was engaged by Dr. Gillig as a site for resident training for the Wright State University Psychiatry Department Community Psychiatry Program, where she teaches and conducts community-based research. This program has been partially funded by the Ohio Department of Mental Health. A Distinguished Fellow of the American Psychiatric Association, Dr. Gillig also has been the Midwestern (Area 4) Representative to the Board of the American Association of Community Psychiatrists and a consultant to the American Psychiatric Association Committee on Poverty, Homelessness, and Psychiatric Disorders. She has been selected as one of the best 3%–5% among doctors in America by Best Doctors, Inc., a Massachusetts-based quality-surveying organization. Dr. Gillig has done clinical work in a variety of settings, including psychiatric emergency services, inpatient state-run psychiatric facilities, Veterans Affairs medical centers, and others. She has completed a doctorate in psychology, a doctorate in medicine, an internal medicine internship, and neurology and psychiatry residencies.

Hunter L. McQuistion, M.D. (editor)

Director, Division of Integrated Psychiatric Services, Department of Psychiatry, The St. Luke's and Roosevelt Hospitals, New York City. Previously, Dr. McQuistion was Chief Medical Officer for Mental Hygiene Services, New York City Department of Health and Mental Hygiene, and Medical Director of Project Renewal, Inc., a New York City nonprofit offering comprehensive care for disabled homeless adults. After gaining his medical degree from the Albany Medical College in Albany, New York, he received his psychiatric training at NYU-Bellevue Medical Center, where he was chief resident. He subsequently completed the Fellowship in Public Psychiatry at the New York State Psychiatric Institute and Columbia University. Dr. McQuistion is Adjunct Associate Clinical Professor of Psychiatry at Mount Sinai School of Medicine and serves on the Voluntary Faculty of the Public Psychiatry Fellowship at the New York State Psychiatric Institute. He has published, presented, and taught on issues in community mental health and the care of underserved populations, especially as they concern advocacy, clinical engagement, psychiatric rehabilitation, substance misuse, and criminal justice. He is also Representative at Large of the American Association of Community Psychiatrists. He is a recipient of the National Alliance on Mental Illness (NAMI) Exemplary Psychiatrist Award, a Fellow of the New York Academy of Medicine, and a Distinguished Fellow of the American Psychiatric Association.

Ralph Aquila, M.D.

Director of Residential Community Service, St. Luke's-Roosevelt Hospital Center, New York City, and Assistant Clinical Professor of Psychiatry, Columbia College of Physicians and Surgeons. The Residential Community Service Program serves about 1,500 persons with serious and persistent mental illness, providing coordination and delivery of medical and psychiatric services to 25 sites in Manhattan. Dr. Aquila is primarily a clinician who works directly with patients who have serious and persistent mental illness, many of whom were formerly homeless. His key focus is the belief in recovery for patients with serious mental illness, which for many persons has been only a dream. Meaningful employment as a psychiatric outcome has become a daily standard in his practice, in coordination with Fountain House, a world-renowned rehabilitation program where he is a consultant. With the advent of new technologies, advocacy, and accountability, the idea of recovery and reintegration is becoming a reality.

Dr. Aquila is chairperson of the Eli Lilly Schizophrenia Scholarship Awards, annual scholarships given to persons with serious and persistent mental illness to obtain or expand their education. He is chairperson of the Eli Lilly Annual Reintegration Awards for persons and programs pursuing reintegration for those with serious and persistent mental illness. He has been Principal Investigator in Stage III atypical antipsychotic drug trials, including olanzapine, ziprasidone, and quetiapine. Most recently, he completed a work outcome study for persons with serious and persistent mental illness that attempts to show a connection between quality psychiatric care and psychiatric rehabilitation. Dr. Aquila currently is Principal Investigator in a cost-effectiveness study to define the cost of treating persons with serious and persistent mental illness. He was a recipient of the 1999 NAMI Exemplary Psychiatrist Award.

Brian D. Bronson, M.D.

Director of Consultation and Liaison Psychiatry and Primary Care Based Mental Health, Veterans Administration New York Harbor Health Care Network, New York Campus, and Clinical Assistant Professor, Department of Psychiatry, New York University School of Medicine. Dr. Bronson completed medical school and residency training at New York University and a dual fellowship in Public Psychiatry at Columbia University and in Consultation and Liaison Psychiatry with specialization in Primary Care at Long Island Jewish–Hillside Medical Center. He also worked in international community psychiatry in Ecuador.

Florence Coleman, M.D.

Chief of Special Emphasis Mental Health Programs, including substance abuse treatment, posttraumatic stress disorder treatment, veterans' industries, health maintenance, and homeless programs, Veterans Affairs Medical Center (VAMC), Dayton, Ohio. Dr. Coleman has served the VAMC for 12 years and is Assistant Professor in the Department of Psychiatry at Wright State University and Assistant Clinical Professor in the Department of Psychiatry of the University of Cincinnati.

Jennifer Dempster, L.P.C.C., L.I.C.D.C.

Site Director, Associate Clinical Director, and Program Supervisor for mental health counselors, Consolidated Care, Inc., Bellefontaine, Ohio. Ms. Dempster has been co-chair of the performance improvement program at Consolidated Care for the last 4 years and supervises the rural domestic violence program, New Directions. She also is involved in many community collaborations such as the Logan County Continuum of Care, the Community Services Management Committee, the Strength-Based Leadership Committee, and the Logan County Triage Committee.

Lisa Dixon, M.D.

Professor of Psychiatry, University of Maryland School of Medicine, and Director of the Division of Services Research in the School's Department of Psychiatry. Dr. Dixon is also the Associate Director for Research of the Veterans Affairs Mental Illness Research, Education and Clinical Center (MIRECC) in VISN5, the Capitol Health Care Network.

Neil Falk, M.D.

Associate Medical Director for Cascadia Behavioral Health Care, Portland, Oregon. Dr. Falk has served the homeless community in Portland for more than 10 years. He also is Adjunct Assistant Professor of Psychiatry at Oregon Health and Sciences University, where he serves as Assistant Director of the Public Psychiatry Training Program.

Alan Felix, M.D.

Medical Director of Project Reachout, providing services to homeless people with mental illness in Manhattan's Upper West Side, and Associate Clinical Professor of Psychiatry, Columbia University College of Physicians and Surgeons, New York. Dr. Felix is one of the developers of the Critical Time Intervention (CTI), an evidence-based model of case management for homeless populations in transition to community-based housing and services. He is the former clinical director of the Westchester Families First program, which utilized Family CTI for homeless families in Westchester County, New York. He is also a consultant to a CTI study of homeless men and women leaving the Bronx and Rockland Psychiatric Centers and to several other CTI applications. Dr. Felix is the former director of the New York Presbyterian Hospital's CTI program in the Fort Washington Armory Shelter in Washington Heights, New York, where he worked for 16 years.

Avrim Fishkind, M.D.

Medical Director of Psychiatric Emergency Services, NeuroPsychiatric Center, Houston, Texas. Dr. Fishkind graduated from the Johns Hopkins Medical School, trained in psychiatry at the Mount Sinai Medical Center in New York City, and finished a fellowship in Public Psychiatry at the New York State Psychiatric Institute. Dr. Fishkind is President-Elect of the American Association for Emergency Psychiatry.

Julie P. Gentile, M.D.

Assistant Professor, Wright State University, Dayton, Ohio. Dr. Gentile is Medical Director at Consumer Advocacy Model, a community agency that serves individuals, including veterans, with mental illness, traumatic brain injury, and substance abuse. She also is project director of the Coordinating Center of Excellence (Mental Illness/Mental Retardation) for the state of Ohio and provides training for community agencies regarding the effective use of multidisciplinary teams, and assessment and management of persons with dual diagnosis. She specializes in the area of dual diagnosis (mental illness and mental retardation) and is the psychiatrist on the multidisciplinary team for the Montgomery County Board of Mental Retardation/Developmental Disabilities.

Stephen M. Goldfinger, M.D.

Dr. Goldfinger is a community psychiatrist whose career has focused on the treatment and rehabilitation of the most seriously disabled psychiatric patients. He is currently Professor and Chair of Psychiatry at the State University of New York, Downstate Medical Center, Brooklyn. He has been Assistant Professor of Psychiatry at Harvard Medical School, the Clinical Director of the Massachusetts Mental Health Center (Harvard's largest public psychiatry program), and the Principal Investigator of a $13 million grant examining models of housing for homeless individuals with serve mental illness. He moved (back home) to New York City in 1997, to Downstate Medical Center, where he "began" his career working in the Department of Psychiatry as a volunteer when he was fifteen!

Dr. Goldfinger is a national expert on homelessness, schizophrenia, and treatment adherence in mental illness. He is the author or editor of over 100 books, monographs, journal articles, and abstracts and is on the editorial boards of numerous publications. He is extremely active in professional organizations and has served as Chair of the APA's Committee on Chronic Mental Illness, Committee on Poverty, Homelessness and Psychiatric Disorders, the Institute on Psychiatric Services, the Committee on Commercial Support, which oversees the relationship between the APA and the pharmaceutical industry, and many subcommittees of the Scientific Program Committee. He is currently vice-chair of the Institute on Psychiatric Services Scientific Program Committee. He is also on the Board of Directors of the American Association of Community Psychiatrists and the Irwin Foundation Recovery Initiative. For almost twenty years, he has served as the volunteer on-site psychiatrist for NAMI's annual convention.

Ann Hackman, M.D.

Assistant Professor of Psychiatry, Director of Community Psychiatry Training and Associate Director of Psychiatry Residency Training, University of Maryland School of Medicine. Dr. Hackman also has been the Medical Director of the Assertive Community Treatment (ACT) Program in Baltimore, Maryland, for over a decade.

John Kelleher

Born in Yonkers, Mr. Kelleher is a native New Yorker who attended Queens College, Hunter College, and the New York University school of visual arts. He has been in recovery from bipolar disorder since the 1960s and currently works full-time as an administrative assistant for St. Luke's-Roosevelt Hospital. He has lectured about his recovery to various audiences and is a recipient of a Lilly Reintegration Award.

H. Richard Lamb, M.D.

Prior to joining the faculty of the University of Southern California, Dr. Lamb worked for the Community Mental Health Services of San Mateo County, California. There, he developed and ran a large vocational rehabilitation service for persons with severe mental illness. In addition, he has run an acute psychiatric inpatient service, a day treatment and aftercare service, and psychiatric emergency services in a large city (Los Angeles). He has been a consultant to probation and police departments. He has also raised money from private sources in order to develop a range of supportive housing for persons with severe mental illness. It was in San Mateo County that Richard met Tony and Fran Hoffman and worked with them to publicize the family movement.

Dr. Lamb has been active with the American Psychiatric Association. He chaired the Task Force on the Homeless Mentally Ill, served twice on the Editorial Board of Psychiatric Services, and was a member of the Committee on Rehabilitation and Vice-Chair of the Council on Psychiatric Services. He chaired the Institute on Psychiatric Services Scientific Program Committee. He currently serves on the Council on Social Issues and Public Psychiatry and the Committee on Jails and Prisons. Dr. Lamb was the recipient of the NAMI 2003 Don and Peggy Richardson Memorial Award for Distinguished Service to Persons Afflicted With Serious Mental Illness. In 1998 he received the American Psychiatric Association's Arnold L. van Ameringen Award in Psychiatric Rehabilitation and Treatment of the Chronically Mentally Ill. Dr. Lamb is currently Professor of Psychiatry and Director of Mental Health Policy and Law at the University of Southern California.

Ann Morrison, M.D.

Director of Community Psychiatry and Associate Professor of Psychiatry, Wright State University, Dayton, Ohio. Dr. Morrison has provided training for the Dayton Veterans Affairs Medical Center about intensive outpatient services and treatment issues such as Program of Assertive Community Treatment (PACT) and outpatient commitment. She is Chief Clinical Officer for the Alcohol, Drug Addiction and Mental Health Services Board for Montgomery County, Ohio. She has provided psychiatric services for PACT teams while in training at the University of Wisconsin, Madison, and with a state-operated program in Montgomery County, as well as a broad range of outpatient and inpatient services in community mental health settings.

David Nardacci, M.D.

Director of Psychiatry and Behavioral Health, Gouverneur Healthcare Services, New York City. Dr. Nardacci is on the faculty at New York University.

Anthony T. Ng, M.D.

Dr. Ng is a psychiatrist with the District of Columbia Department of Mental Health and with Health Care for the Homeless in Baltimore, Maryland. He is on the faculty of the Uniformed Services School of Medicine, George Washington University School of Medicine, and the New York University School of Nursing. He received his bachelor's degree at the City College of New York and his medical degree at SUNY at Buffalo School of Medicine and completed his psychiatry residency at St. Vincent's Hospital in New York City. He was a Public Psychiatry Fellow at Columbia/Presbyterian Hospital. He has given many lectures and conferences on cultural competency, disaster mental health, and homelessness outreach. He was formerly the Medical Director of Disaster Psychiatry Outreach and Associate Medical Director of Project Renewal, Inc., a not-for-profit organization serving the adult homeless population of New York City.

Fred Osher, M.D.

Director, Center for Behavioral Health, Justice, and Public Policy, and Associate Professor of Psychiatry, University of Maryland School of Medicine. Dr. Osher is a community psychiatrist with clinical, research, and policy interests focusing on the co-occurrence of mental and substance use disorders. Over the last two decades, he has led clinical and research efforts for persons with these disorders within our community settings, increasingly in our jails and prisons, and in populations without adequate housing. He has a long history of public-sector service at local, state, and federal levels. Previous positions include Director of Community Psychiatry at the University of Maryland; Acting Director of the Division of Demonstration Programs at the Center for Mental Health Services, Substance Abuse and Mental Health Services Administration; and Deputy Director of the Office of Programs for the Homeless Mentally Ill at the National Institute of Mental Health. Dr. Osher has published extensively and provided comprehensive training in the areas of homelessness, community psychiatry, co-occurring mental and addictive disorders, and effective approaches to persons with behavioral disorders who have contact with the criminal justice system.

Elizabeth Oudens, M.D.

Director of Psychiatric Services for Project Renewal, a not-for-profit organization in New York City providing comprehensive rehabilitative services for homeless and formerly homeless individuals. Dr. Oudens previously served for 3 years as Medical Director of Project Renewal's Fort Washington Shelter for homeless mentally ill men. Dr. Oudens is a graduate of the Columbia University Public Psychiatry Fellowship. She attended medical school and psychiatry residency at the University of California, San Francisco, where she was one of the co-founders of the student-run medical clinic for the homeless.

Anne M. Piette, L.M.S.W.

Senior Social Worker at St. Vincent's Hospital, Manhattan, in the Department of Community Medicine, SRO/Homeless. Ms. Piette received her bachelor of arts degree from Rhode Island College in 1975. From 1976 to 1981 she was a caseworker at Blackstone Valley Regional Center, Rhode Island. She received her master's degree in social work in 1983 at Columbia University, and her certification in social work in 1984. From 1983 to 1990, she was an Outreach Team Leader for Project Renewal in New York City.

Erik Roskes, M.D.

Director of Forensic Treatment, Springfield Hospital Center, Sykesville, Maryland. Dr. Roskes has long been interested in the complex problems facing individuals with mental illness involved in the criminal justice system. He maintains an active outpatient practice working with individuals who are court mandated to participate in mental health treatment as a condition of their release to community settings. Additionally, he serves as a Compliance Monitor in *Brad H. et al v. City of New York et al,* a case involving the provision of transition planning to jail detainees and inmates leaving the New York jail system and returning to their communities. As a consultant to the Council of State Governments, he provides technical assistance to jurisdictions across the country working on developing criminal justice/mental health collaborations. Previously, Dr. Roskes served as Chief Psychiatrist in the Maryland Department of Public Safety and Correctional Services.

Judith Samuels, Ph.D.

Head, Policy Analytic Lab, and Research Scientist, Nathan Kline Institute for Psychiatric Research. She is the Principal Investigator of a study funded by the Substance Abuse and Mental Health Services Administration, "The Impact of the Family Critical Time Intervention on Homeless Children." Dr. Samuels also is the project manager for SAMHSA's NYC Housing Alternative Initiative for persons with serious mental illness and a member of that study's cross-site steering committee. The experimental program for homeless families developed under Dr. Samuels' direction is cited as a model program in President Bush's New Freedom Commission on Mental Health final report, *Achieving the Promise: Transforming Mental Health Care in America.* Dr. Samuels' research has focused on areas related to mental health, public policy, and homeless populations.

Randie Schacter, D.O.

Dr. Schacter is a practicing child and adolescent psychiatrist, on staff at Presbyterian Hospital, Charlotte, North Carolina. A graduate of the New York College of Osteopathic Medicine, She completed her training in General Psychiatry and Child & Adolescent Psychiatry at the North Shore Long Island Jewish Health System, New York. She has received the American Academy of Child and Adolescent Psychiatry Outstanding Resident Award and the New York College of Osteopathic Medicine Presidential Service Award.

Manoj Shah, M.D.

Director, Child and Adolescent Psychiatry, Brookdale University Hospital and Medical Center, and in private practice, Dr. Shah is the former medical director of the Recognition and Prevention Program in the Division of Child and Adolescent Psychiatry, Schneider Children's/Zucker Hillside Hospital, North Shore-Long Island System, New Hyde Park, New York. He is a board certified child and adolescent psychiatrist and is Assistant Professor of Psychiatry at the Albert Einstein College of Medicine in New York City. He is a Fellow of the American Academy of Child and Adolescent Psychiatry, a Distinguished Fellow of the American Psychiatric Association, an Honorary Fellow of the Indian Psychiatric Society, and a Fellow of the Royal College of Psychiatrists, United Kingdom.

Thomas Sweet

Mr. Sweet has worked at Fountain House in New York City for over 20 years and is currently Director of Planning. He works with the president, the board of directors, the research director, and the membership on strategic planning, designing, developing, and launching new initiatives, and optimizing Fountain House systems and operations. He also has authored grants, primarily for funding from governmental sources, that provide operational money for various programs and projects at Fountain House. He currently serves as the Chief Information Officer and also supervises the Management Information Services department.

Scott Zeller, M.D.

Chief of Psychiatric Emergency Services, Alameda County Medical Center, Oakland, California. Dr. Zeller graduated from Northwestern University Medical School and trained in psychiatry at the University of California, San Francisco. He is the Western Regional Director of the American Association for Emergency Psychiatry.

ACKNOWLEDGMENTS

We thank Harry Newton and Francis Greenburger for their generous support in the publication of this book. We are very grateful as well to Bristol-Myers Squibb and the American Psychiatric Foundation. Finally, we thank Larry Gillig for his unflagging enthusiasm, support, and encouragement for this project.

FOREWORD

When the American Psychiatric Association's first Task Force on the Homeless Mentally Ill made its recommendations (Talbott and Lamb 1984), we thought we were well on the way to resolving the problems of persons with severe mental illness who are homeless. When the American Psychiatric Association's second Task Force made its report eight years later (Lamb et al. 1992), we found that we had acquired considerably more knowledge about the nature of the problem and possible solutions, but we were disappointed that so little had been accomplished to actually reduce homelessness in this population.

Again, we made a series of recommendations. First of all, we strongly endorsed the recommendations of the first Task Force and encouraged the launching of wide-scale efforts to implement them. Because so little had been done, we emphasized that the treatment and rehabilitation of persons with severe mental illness must be made the highest priority in public mental health and receive the first priority for public funding. Such efforts would of course include those who are homeless or at risk of becoming homeless.

We pointed out the need for a range of treatment interventions encompassing both community and hospital alternatives. Thus, many individuals able to live in the community may, at times of crisis, require more intensive support and structure. We pointed out that community workers serving severely mentally ill persons who are homeless must receive training in the recognition and assessment of both functional strengths and dangerous degrees of disability. We emphasized the need for a practical approach based on clinical reality and emphasized that those who served homeless, severely mentally ill persons must neither glorify autonomy nor dismiss individual rights; the individual in need must be given access to appropriate care.

We noted that it is frequently said that homeless mentally ill individuals live on the streets by choice. We further noted, however, that this is an allegation that flies in the face of both clinical observation and research data, for the reality is that life on the streets is generally characterized by dysphoria and extreme deprivation. It often leads to victimization by the human predators of the streets and very frequently precipitates the onset of life-threatening medical problems. It had already been clearly demonstrated that many, though by no means all, severely mentally ill homeless individuals will voluntarily accept an offer of safe and supportive housing.

Now, fourteen years later, this new clinical guide is very much needed. First of all, it is heartening to know that there are dedicated persons who continue both to work with and to write about persons with severe mental illness who are homeless. What is needed are successful efforts to conceptualize the nature and cause of the problem and then develop a practical clinical guide. That is what these authors have accomplished.

Workers in the field need to know the practicalities of how to do outreach and engage homeless mentally ill persons in both urban and rural settings; the importance of providing high-quality supportive and therapeutic housing; and how to help homeless single adults, families and children, and homeless veterans. Workers need to know how to set up and run mobile crisis teams and assertive community treatment, and they need to know what is involved in the emergency psychiatric treatment of homeless persons, both on the streets and in emergency rooms. There are specific ways that psychiatric inpatient treatment can set the stage for a successful rehabilitation of severely mentally ill homeless persons, and these need to be spelled out. Primary care staff as well as mental health staff have important roles to play with this population, but first, practical guidelines are needed.

Frequently, severely mentally ill persons shuttle back and forth between the streets and jails or prisons. This problem needs to be addressed, and it is addressed in this volume. No problem is more important than this one.

It is my hope that the availability of this new guide to clinical care will greatly increase society's efforts to take meaningful action to help persons with severe mental illness who are homeless.

H. Richard Lamb, M.D.

REFERENCES

Lamb HR, Bachrach LL, Kass FI (eds): Treating the Homeless Mentally Ill: A Task Force Report of the American Psychiatric Association. Washington, DC, American Psychiatric Association, 1992

Talbott JA, Lamb HR: Summary and recommendations, in The Homeless Mentally Ill: A Task Force Report of the American Psychiatric Association. Edited by Lamb HR. Washington, DC, American Psychiatric Association, 1984, pp 1–10

Chapter 1

MENTAL ILLNESS AND HOMELESSNESS

An Introduction

Hunter L. McQuistion, M.D.
Paulette Marie Gillig, M.D., Ph.D.

We have set out to assemble a practical clinical guide for work with homeless people who have mental illness, written *by clinicians, for clinicians*. It approaches treatment and rehabilitation from the vantage point of the treatment environment, from street to housing—and, we hope, almost everything in between.

The ideas in this book reflect what we believe is the evolution of consensus on a clinical approach to the homeless mentally ill person, developed over more than two decades by many experts but until now not assembled in a detailed, practical format. Over the years, the experts contributing to this consensus have been both academic and frontline—and, especially in the beginning, they have been volunteer clinicians who built this knowledge when they were often the only resource for homeless people. Although the focus of this clinical guide is psychiatric, psychiatrists have joined with other mental health and chemical dependency professionals and with formerly homeless peer workers in developing the techniques described here. Gathering this evolving body of knowledge is a multidisciplinary process—simply because the complexity of the social and clinical problems involved in work with homeless patients demands collaboration.

AN EVOLVING CONSENSUS

Consensual evolution implies development. The mental health and substance abuse service system has developed in sophistication—although obviously this has not resulted in the disappearance of homelessness in America, which has persisted as a structural economic, social, and political problem. But there has also been the exciting ascendance of the consumer as an active guide in his and her own mental health services planning, helping the clinician solve homelessness "one patient at a time." It is often said that the clinical innovations developed through work with homeless populations have influenced practice with those who have serious psychiatric disorders but are domiciled. Providers of homelessness services have historically placed an emphasis on meeting manifest needs and personal goals. This emphasis on needs and goals, as well as the utilization of peer workers, has now placed clinicians who work with homeless populations in the vanguard of understanding for emerging models of recovery in mental health services (American Association of Community Psychiatrists 2003).

Recovery and the clinical interventions that serve it are pieces of a much broader effort to end homelessness. This has not always been a point of full agreement. Earlier in the now-endemic wave of latter-day American homelessness, there was debate about the role of mental health care, with polarized views on whether it was needed at all versus whether housing was even possible without it. The early 1990s brought a greater understanding of the epidemiology of homelessness (Susser et al. 1993), and this debate among advocates was largely resolved. A clear understanding emerged that those with psychiatric disorders, including chemical dependence, need aggressive and integrated psychiatric rehabilitation to succeed, but that access to housing is prerequisite to anything else.

Studies show reasonably consistent rates among homeless people of one-third to one-half with severe psychiatric disorders, whether major mood disorder (20%–30%) or schizophrenia (10%–15%) (Breakey et al. 1989; Koegel et al. 1988; Roth et al; 1985; Susser et al. 1989). Rates of substance and alcohol abuse were reported as 20%–30% and 57%–63%, respectively (Fischer et al. 1986; Koegel et al. 1988; Vernez et al. 1988). Mental health needs of homeless people are documented as far back as 1969 (Spitzer et al. 1969). Set in the context of deinstitutionalization, Lamb's *The Homeless Mentally Ill* (1984) was a landmark. The first major work focusing on this population, it concentrated on causation and intervention systems and contained glimmers of a clinical approach, most notably on the roles of interdisciplinary support, continuous relationships and case management, hospitalization, neurobiological features, and medical needs (Brickner et al. 1984; Drake and Adler 1984; Kaufmann 1984; Goldfinger and Chafetz 1984; Lipton and Sabatini 1984).

As pioneering mental health professionals began to work with mentally ill homeless people, clinical challenges and approaches became more defined. Breakey (1987) identified barriers to treatment. In addition to discussing the patent issues of housing, service access, and the "ubiquity of alcohol,"

Breakey described how disaffiliation, distrust and disenchantment, mobility, and the multiplicity of clinical and social needs mark homelessness. Of these, disaffiliation (Bahr 1970), an alienated existential state marked by attenuation or absence of relationships, is a defining challenge to clinicians, who must establish a meaningful relationship in order to offer assistance. Not surprisingly, the authors of our guide examine the process of therapeutic engagement in detail and from multiple angles.

Susser and colleagues (1990) described a psychiatrist who ran a weekly bingo game in a shelter as a means of overcoming fear, stigma, and alienation, a nonthreatening device to form relationships. They also highlighted the technique of purposeful "chatting" to build trust, recognizing it as an implicit acceptance of a need for help. Chatting builds a critical empathic bridge toward creating a shared therapeutic language with the potential patient (McQuistion et al. 1991). Furthermore, through their experiences, Susser and colleagues also importantly noted that healing occurs in a social context. Homeless populations are encountered in a range of settings, and clinical interventions must attune themselves to the culture and subcultures in which they are embedded. Our agreement with this observation influences the setting-specific format of this book.

Though detailed discussion is beyond this book's scope, social context also includes understanding how cultural identity influences human experience and behavior (Lim 2006). Basic clinical competence requires mental health professionals to actively integrate issues concerning race, ethnicity, gender, and sexual orientation into their work. Relating to our patients through this lens enables us to build an empathic bridge to engagement, and then to healing. It is a particularly poignant issue for homeless individuals, whose disaffiliation can be exacerbated by racial and other culturally based marginalizing attitudes.

After editing his first book on homelessness and mental illness, Lamb co-edited an equally influential sequel, *Treating the Homeless Mentally Ill* (Lamb et al. 1992), which began to lay down principles of treatment and rehabilitation, identifying and discussing integral service components such as co-occurring chemical dependency (Minkoff and Drake 1992), social skills (Vaccaro et al. 1992), and residential programming (Bebout and Harris 1992).

This volume also began to discuss experiential challenges in working with this population (Chafetz 1992), opening the clinically important issue of countertransference in work with homeless patients. Surprisingly, this topic is not frequently written about in detail. Countertransference issues in this setting are typically related to the "otherness" of our own usually more benign backgrounds. Working with homeless people's destitution, disaffiliation, and often intensely traumatic histories normatively activates within us strong emotions that include anxiety, guilt, anger, and depression. Conversely, it can also evoke unrealistic optimism. These feelings can provoke clinicians to excessive coercion, therapeutic withdrawal, and idealized expectations. They can also yield boundary challenges beyond the real object orientation necessary in working with this population as, for example, in lending personal funds to an impoverished patient. The maintenance of empathy requires self-examination and the psychological growth that accompanies it (Felix and Wine 2001; Ng and McQuistion 2004), a process that both complements and helps develop the cultural competence we describe above. This process can also help clinicians learn how to be mutually supportive in difficult treatment environments.

A STRUCTURE FOR REHABILITATION

Another especially important contribution of Lamb and colleagues' book was its proposal of theoretical scaffolding on which to build rehabilitation (Susser et al. 1992), linking stages of intervention to the trajectory of a homeless person from street to housing. As long as it is sufficiently flexible and contemporaneously relevant to the service system, such a structure is useful to clinicians as they weigh the nature, intensity, sequence, and timing of their interventions.

As described in detail elsewhere (McQuistion et al. 2003a), one of the editors of this clinical guide endeavored to develop this structure, describing three essential phases of rehabilitation: engagement, intensive care, and ongoing rehabilitation.

- **Engagement** is the first phase, in which clinicians build a relationship, using it as leverage to offer help of any kind.
- **Intensive care** augurs a necessarily multidisciplinary process of collaborative goal setting with the patient concerning entitlements and housing access, in which medical, substance abuse, and mental health interventions are approached. This stage may also involve vocational and social rehabilitative aspects.
- **Ongoing rehabilitation** is an open-ended stage in which the patient establishes an identity as no longer homeless and moves to another phase of recovery, such as the reestablishment of family ties.

As you use this clinical guide, we hope that knowledge of this structure will help in your conceptualization of the site-specific material. Treatment setting or specific subpopulation organizes this guide. We expect that you will turn to the chapters most relevant to your work or areas of interest or teaching and learning (McQuistion et al. 2004). However, the guide does have an organizational logic in that the next five chapters follow a sequence of naturalistic settings, in which first engagement, then intensive care, and finally ongoing rehabilitation take place. The last eight chapters define specific, and in most cases more formal, treatment settings that interact with patients at various points on the continuum from engagement to ongoing rehabilitation. Each chapter is case-based and accompanied by a service flowchart. In addition to describing the unique features and services of the setting, each chapter covers diagnosis, treatment planning, and access to entitlements.

A STEP IN THE EVOLUTION OF "BEST PRACTICES"

Finally, we view this clinical guide as an evolutionary step itself. The epidemiology of homelessness continues to change (McQuistion et al. 2003b; North 2004) and therefore, so will service needs. As of our writing in late 2005, we witness a special national emphasis on ending chronic homelessness (U.S. Interagency Council on Homelessness 2005) and the affirmation of housing as indispensable. Indeed, "housing-first" models, which emphasize rapid transitional or permanent supportive housing, bypassing or truncating classic shelter stays, arguably show great promise in fostering hope and reducing demoralization among people who are homeless and have psychiatric disorders (Tsemberis and Eisenberg 2000). As described in Chapter 5 of the guide, Assertive Community Treatment (ACT) is integral to many of these housing models and holds credibility as an evidence-based intervention. Similarly, as described in the chapter on homeless families (Chapter 4), Critical Time Intervention (CTI) is another practice supported by increasingly accumulating data. Moreover, on an essentially practical level, any program intervention using the clinical and rehabilitative techniques herein described is ripe for continuous quality improvement methodology. Community-based mental health care, especially in nontraditional settings, has lagged in methodically evaluating and improving effectiveness.

With new and constantly evolving practices in mind, the next step for the material such as exists in this manual would be further elaboration and translation to best practices. In the report *Blueprint for Change* (2003), the federal Substance Abuse and Mental Health Services Administration identified essential systemic service components, pointing to practices and tenets to guide the construction of services for this population. Having an analogous set of best clinical practices would be as useful for the clinician as the *Blueprint* is for the policymaker.

REFERENCES

American Association of Community Psychiatrists: Findings: position statement on recovery-oriented services. AACP, 2003. Available at: http://www.comm.psych.pitt.edu/finds/ROSMenu.html Accessed December 10, 2005.

Bahr HM: Disaffiliated Man: Essays and Bibliography on Skid Row, Vagrancy, and Outsiders. Toronto, ON, Canada, University of Toronto Press, 1970

Bebout RR, Harris M: In search of pumpkin shells: residential programming for the homeless mentally ill, in Treating the Homeless Mentally Ill: A Task Force Report of the American Psychiatric Association. Edited by Lamb HR, Bachrach LL, Kass FI. Washington, DC, American Psychiatric Association, 1992, pp 159–182

Breakey WR: Treating the homeless. Alcohol Health Res World 11:42–47, 1987

Breakey WR, Fischer PJ, Kramer M, et al: Health and mental health problems of homeless men and women in Baltimore. JAMA 262:1352–1357, 1989

Brickner PW, Filardo T, Iseman M, et al: Medical aspects of homelessness, in The Homeless Mentally Ill: A Task Force Report of the American Psychiatric Association. Edited by Lamb HR. Washington, DC, American Psychiatric Association, 1984, pp 243–260

Chafetz L: Why clinicians distance themselves from the homeless mentally ill, in Treating the Homeless Mentally Ill: A Task Force Report of the American Psychiatric Association. Edited by Lamb HR, Bachrach LL, Kass FI. Washington, DC, American Psychiatric Association, 1992, pp 95–108

Drake RE, Adler DA: Shelter is not enough: clinical work with the homeless mentally ill, in The Homeless Mentally Ill: A Task Force Report of the American Psychiatric Association. Edited by Lamb HR. Washington, DC, American Psychiatric Association, 1984, pp 141–152

Felix AD, Wine PR: From the couch to the street: applications of psychoanalysis to work with individuals who are homeless and mentally ill. Journal of Applied Psychoanalytic Studies 3:17–32, 2001

Fischer PJ, Shapiro S, Breakey WR, et al: Mental health and social characteristics of the homeless: a survey of mission users. Am J Public Health 76:519–524, 1986

Goldfinger SM, Chafetz L: Developing a better service system for the homeless mentally ill, in The Homeless Mentally Ill: A Task Force Report of the American Psychiatric Association. Edited by Lamb HR. Washington, DC, American Psychiatric Association, 1984, pp 91–108

Kaufmann CA: Implications of biological psychiatry for the severely mentally ill: a highly vulnerable population, in The Homeless Mentally Ill: A Task Force Report of the American Psychiatric Association. Edited by Lamb HR, Washington, DC, American Psychiatric Association, 1984, pp 201–242

Koegel P, Burnam MA, Farr RK: The prevalence of specific psychiatric disorders among homeless individuals in the inner city of Los Angeles. Arch Gen Psychiatry 45:1085–1092, 1988

Lamb HR (ed): The Homeless Mentally Ill: A Task Force Report of the American Psychiatric Association. Washington, DC, American Psychiatric Association, 1984

Lamb HR, Bachrach LL, Kass FI (eds): Treating the Homeless Mentally Ill: A Task Force Report of the American Psychiatric Association. Washington, DC, American Psychiatric Association, 1992

Lim RF (ed): Clinical Manual of Cultural Psychiatry. Washington, DC, American Psychiatric Publishing, 2006

Lipton FR, Sabatini A: Constructing support systems for chronic patients, in The Homeless Mentally Ill: A Task Force Report of the American Psychiatric Association. Edited by Lamb HR. Washington, DC, American Psychiatric Association, 1984, pp 153–172

McQuistion HL, D'Ercole A, Kopelson E: Urban street outreach: using clinical principles to steer the system. New Dir Ment Health Serv Winter(52):17–27, 1991

McQuistion HL, Felix A, Susser ES: Serving homeless people with mental illness, in Psychiatry, 2nd Edition. Edited by Tasman A, Lieberman J, Kay J. London, Wiley, 2003a, pp 2314–2321

McQuistion HL, Finnerty M, Hirschowitz J, et al: Challenges for psychiatry in serving homeless people with psychiatric disorders. Psychiatr Serv 54:669–676, 2003b

McQuistion HL, Ranz JM, Gillig PM: A survey of American psychiatric residency programs concerning education in homelessness. Acad Psychiatry 28:116–121, 2004

Minkoff K, Drake RE: Homelessness and dual diagnosis, in Treating the Homeless Mentally Ill: A Task Force Report of the American Psychiatric Association. Edited by Lamb HR, Bachrach LL, Kass FI. Washington, DC, American Psychiatric Association, 1992, pp 221–247

Ng AT, McQuistion HL: Outreach to the homeless: craft, science, and future implications. J Psychiatr Pract 10:95–105, 2004

North CS, Eyrich KM, Pollio DE, et al: Are rates of psychiatric disorders in the homeless population changing? Am J Public Health 94:103–108, 2004

Roth D, Bean GJ, Lust N, et al: Homelessness in Ohio: A Study of People in Need. Columbus, Ohio Department of Mental Health, 1985

Spitzer RL, Cohen G, Miller JD, et al: The psychiatric status of 100 men on skid row. Int J Soc Psychiatry 15:230–234, 1969

Substance Abuse and Mental Health Services Administration: Blueprint for Change: Ending Chronic Homelessness for Persons with Serious Mental Illnesses and Co-Occurring Substance Use Disorders (DHHS Publ No SMA-04–3870). Rockville, MD, Center for Mental Health Services, Substance Abuse and Mental Health Services Administration, 2003

Susser E, Struening EL, Conover S: Psychiatric problems in homeless men: lifetime psychosis, substance use, and current distress in new arrivals at New York City shelters. Arch Gen Psychiatry 46:845–850, 1989

Susser ES, Goldfinger SM, White A: Some clinical approaches to the homeless mentally ill. Community Ment Health J 26:463–480, 1990

Susser ES, Valencia E, Goldfinger SM: Clinical care of homeless mentally ill individuals: strategies and adaptations, in Treating the Homeless Mentally Ill: A Task Force Report of the American Psychiatric Association. Edited by Lamb HR, Bachrach LL, Kass FI. Washington, DC, American Psychiatric Association, 1992, pp 127–140

Susser E, Valencia E, Conover S: Prevalence of HIV infection among psychiatric patients in a New York City men's shelter Am J Public Health 83:568–570, 1993

Tsemberis S, Eisenberg RF: Pathways to housing: supported housing for street-dwelling homeless individuals with psychiatric disabilities. Psychiatr Serv 51:487–493, 2000

U.S. Interagency Council on Homelessness: State and Local Information. Available at: http://www.ich.gov/slocal/index.html. Accessed December 11, 2005.

Vaccaro JV, Liberman RP, Friedlob S, Dempsay S: Challenge and opportunity: rehabilitating the homeless mentally ill, in Treating the Homeless Mentally Ill: A Task Force Report of the American Psychiatric Association. Edited by Lamb HR, Bachrach LL, Kass FI. Washington, DC, American Psychiatric Association, 1992, pp 279–298

Vernez G, Burnam MA, McGlynn EA, et al: Review of California's Program for the Homeless Mentally Disabled. Santa Monica, CA, Rand Corporation, 1988

Chapter 2

GENERAL CONCEPTS OF OUTREACH AND ENGAGEMENT

Neil Falk, M.D.

PREPARING FOR ACTIVE TREATMENT

Establishing a Community Presence

> Mark is a 32-year-old man initially encountered while he was living in a garbage collection station under a freeway overpass. When approached by an outreach team, he refused contact, either walking away or yelling at the team to leave him alone. After continued failed attempts at verbal contact, the team began leaving food and cigarettes near his dumpster. After a few weeks, Mark began asking the team for "food and smokes," and soon he began briefly speaking with them. After 4 months, he agreed to meet with the team's psychiatrist.

Working with homeless mentally ill individuals requires using a different template from that available in more traditional services. This difference is exemplified in how clients enter treatment. In the traditional setting, a client is often directed toward a provider by an insurer, word of mouth, or referral from a primary care provider. Each of these approaches implies that mental health services are available and are acceptable not only to the client, but to the community at large. However, among homeless people, mental health care is often viewed as at best a luxury or at worst, a declaration of vulnerability.

Accordingly, the first goal of treating homeless mentally ill people must be establishing oneself as acceptable to homeless people (Morse et al. 1996). As is often the theme in such work, this entails providing the client, in this case the population as a whole, with what it wants. Therefore, mental health care providers must be viewed as working toward the goals of the homeless—obtaining the basic needs of food, clothing, shelter, and companionship. Although first stabilizing mental illness may achieve these goals more consistently and permanently for a minority of clients, this approach generally results in failure, because clients' motivations are to obtain basic needs such as food, shelter, safety, transportation, education, medical treatment, and vocational services (Acosta and Toro 2000).

Many clients are also estranged from the entire homeless services community. These are clients who refuse organized systems of care and remain on the street, without formal shelter. These clients need gentle outreach efforts to help them gain trust in mental health providers. In our experience, many of these clients are psychotically paranoid or otherwise mistrustful and must be allowed to dictate the pace of establishing rapport. In some cases, it may be years before a therapeutic alliance is established. Although this lengthy process can frustrate the provider, hastening the process may be alienating. Meeting the client's identified needs while slowly introducing the team's goals will best allow progress toward engaging the client in treatment (Morse et al. 1996).

Engagement

Because homeless people often will not identify themselves as needing mental health services, mental health workers must count on other community resources to identify potential clients. Two goals must be accomplished to create good referral sources. One is to make the mental health system available to the referral sources in a way that helps them meet their goals. For example, offering more permanent housing resources through a mental health center helps other community members understand that the mental health team is effective and reliable. The second goal is to respond to acute mental health issues. Responding to these issues offers support and safety to community residents, business owners, and police officers, all of whom interact with homeless individuals. After a team has proved to community stakeholders that it is attentive and effective, those same groups will reply in kind, creating a comprehensive care network (Rowe et al. 1998).

Once a client is identified, the team must instill the value of treatment and rehabilitation in the client. As noted earlier, at this stage clients are primarily working toward survival, and engagement must meet these needs while simultaneously establishing rapport. If these two goals are met, introducing mental health care is more likely to succeed (Park et al. 2002). Successful strategies must include offering clients help with identifying sources of food (soup kitchens, food giveaways), housing (shelters, drop-in centers, supportive apartments), and clothing (shelters, charities). In addition, clients value comforts—such as cigarettes, coffee, socks, and blankets—and importantly, educational and vocational opportunities.

Once engagement has reached the point of introducing mental health care, the team often employs harm reduction and motivational interviewing techniques (Miller et al. 2002), with a "stages of change" clinical model (Prochaska et al. 1994) to help the client identify symptoms and the ways in which they prevent him or her from reaching goals. In essence, these techniques allow clients to work at their own pace with nonjudgmental support from staff, and they provide staff with a theoretical framework and tools with which to reach clients. Once the client agrees that an issue exists, he or she can be moved toward intensive treatment as part of its solution.

ACTIVE TREATMENT

> Mark agreed to meet the outreach team's psychiatrist at the clinic, but only with promises of some food and the presence of a team member at the interview. He noted that he was living in the garbage collection center to avoid people, as they generally bothered and harassed him. He also complained that women often accused him of making sexually inappropriate comments, which he attributed to their "lack of a sense of humor." He initially saw no reason to start medications, denying classic symptoms of mental illness (despite displaying paranoid and religious delusions, responses to internal stimuli, disorganized thinking, and thought blocking), but requested to meet regularly with the psychiatrist to "talk about his life and figure out his spiritual mission." He refused to sign up for entitlements, out of fear that the information "would be sent to the government and used against him." He eventually accepted antipsychotic medication after 3 months of regular contact, although sample medications were used because Mark had no entitlements. He experienced significant improvement in his psychotic symptoms, and after a few months he agreed to apply for entitlements.

The temptation to rush into symptom management strategies is strong. However, the goal of early treatment must be to establish a foundation for future ongoing treatment, and early treatment emphasizes data gathering and establishment of entitlements. Much clinical information has likely been gathered during the initial engagement period, but demographic and historical data must be collected as well.

Once an adequate database has been established, applications may be completed to obtain entitlements. In addition, the client must agree to the application process. Psychiatric symptoms often interfere with this level of necessary collaboration, owing to paranoia, apathy, depression, disorganization, and agoraphobia, among other factors. Also challenging are denial of symptoms or of needs and a common mistrust of institutional authority.

The most common and essential benefits are Supplemental Security Income (SSI) or Social Security Disability Insurance (SSDI), Medicaid, Medicare, and housing. SSI/SSDI applications are made through the local federal Social Security Administration (SSA) office. In general, applications for these benefits can go through two or three rounds of review and appeal; they usually take a minimum of 3 months to process but can take up to 3 years. When SSI/SSDI is granted, clients generally also receive a payment retroactive to the date of their initial application and become eligible for Medicare. While awaiting the completion of this process, clients can simultaneously apply for and receive state-administered benefits, such as Medicaid and public assistance. Persons with disabilities are among the groups that qualify for Medicaid. The speed at which Medicaid is granted varies according to locality, but the process generally takes a few weeks or months.

Unfortunately, these processes are not well coordinated and may place people with disabilities in a difficult situation. Unless the client is at least 65, he or she will not receive Medicare until 2 years after SSI/SSDI is granted. Furthermore, clients often obtain Medicaid while awaiting the decision on their application for SSI/SSDI. Once granted, SSI/SSDI's income levels (in 2006, $603 per month for an individual receiving SSI and a higher amount based on work history for those receiving SSDI) may disqualify people in some states from Medicaid eligibility unless they can provide proof of certain medically related expenses that help them "spend down" to local Medicaid income eligibility levels. In addition, the insurance later provided under Medicare often carries fewer benefits than Medicaid, forcing some into choosing between adequate medical care with no income and lesser insurance with a small net income.

Some states and localities allocate funding for capital development and program expenses for supportive housing. However, housing entitlements are generally provided by the federal government through the Department of Housing and Urban Development (HUD) but administered locally by various organizations. These benefits generally consist of rent subsidies/vouchers (provided through the Section 8 Tenant Based Assistance: Housing Choice Voucher Program) and are based on financial need (Code of Federal Regulations 2005). This system allows voucher holders to pay a percentage of their income as their rental payment, with HUD paying the remainder of the fair-market rent set by a landlord. In most urban locations, applications for such vouchers are accepted for only a short period once per year. Applicants enter into a pool from which some are chosen randomly every 18–48 months to receive vouchers. There are restrictions in the type of housing and the number of people in each unit, and waiting periods for applicants can extend to 2 to 3 years.

Successful entitlements application obviously requires the establishment of trust, which outreach workers hope to obtain during engagement. However, some clients may need an additional benefit of psychotropic medication to decrease symptoms and allow for this level of rapport. Thus, an intensive amalgam of ongoing engagement, data gathering, social work, and biologic treatments coexist for some. Because rapport may be tentative at this time, an adverse response to medications may destroy this amalgam and result in a rehabilitation setback. The introduction of medication in a fashion favoring tolerability is usually the most effective.

Unfortunately, at this stage psychopharmacological treatment is often tenuously stable. Adherence is often poor because clients have difficulty tracking appointments, remembering medication doses, and holding on to their belongings. One effective approach to improve adherence is to help the client establish a physical or psychological routine and a home base. This milieu can take many forms, the best of which is stable housing (McQuistion et al. 2003; Sullivan et al. 2000). This will allow a reliable location for meetings, a safe environment to store belongings, a central location in which to leave messages, and a base for the client to exist in. Lesser alternatives include a "squat," a routine meeting place (either in a clinic or in the community), or simply the knowledge that the outreach team will always be at a certain place at a certain time, for example at a weekly food giveaway site or every morning at a soup kitchen. Without such a base, the risk of treatment failure is high.

Somatic Health Issues

Mark quickly obtained a small income through a local benefit plan and after 2 months agreed to move into single-room-occupancy housing. However, he became symptomatic within a month of moving in and began harassing his neighbors because of his paranoid delusions. The team believed this was due to Mark's increased alcohol use after entering housing: likely a response to the increased stress of community living, leading to decreased adherence, then recurrent psychosis. As his alcohol use continued, he developed gastritis, the symptoms of which he attributed to his neighbor "injecting him through the wall with CIA medication" while he slept. After Mark's harassment of this neighbor escalated, he was evicted. He was psychiatrically hospitalized a few weeks later when he presented to a local emergency room for medical attention.

Both homelessness and mental illness increase the risk of somatic health concerns (Gelberg et al. 1990; Scott 1993). However, mentally ill homeless individuals seek care for physical illnesses less often (Desai et al. 2003), even though they often are more likely to receive medical benefits (Sullivan et al. 2000) than their domiciled counterparts. Common concerns include parasitic skin infections, abscesses, upper respiratory and urinary tract infections, untreated chronic illnesses such as diabetes mellitus, hypertension, and chronic obstructive pulmonary disease, and both acute and chronic pain syndromes.

Often overlooked is dental pathology, including caries, periodontal disease, excessively mobile teeth, and lack of teeth or dentures (Waplington et al. 2000). These maladies have a range of effects, varying from pain-associated increases in psychiatric symptoms to malnutrition and dehydration.

When a person is living on the street, the care of somatic illness can be even more challenging than psychiatric treatment. In such an uncontrolled environment, arriving at a correct diagnosis is exceedingly difficult without the availability of specialized mobile medical services focusing on the care of the street homeless (Nuttbrock et al. 2003). The psychiatrist's primary role in such circumstances is often that of watchful waiting, persuasion, and facilitating linkage to medical services. The urgency with which to address somatic health needs depends on many factors, including levels of rapport and severity of illness. The severity of symptoms is often recognized by the client and can be used as an actual incentive to engage with the outreach team. However, the client may prioritize his or her needs differently than the psychiatrist, often minimizing the severity of (or denying the presence of) physical illness. These issues must be balanced with an eye to the holistic care of the client. Medical illnesses may progress to the point of needing emergency attention. This may necessitate the placement of an involuntary measure, which risks the erosion of many months of rapport building and engagement work. The following example illustrates many of these issues.

> Sharon appeared to be in her mid-50s and was well known to the outreach team from frequent brief contacts. She was routinely friendly but refused all offers of help from the team, preferring to sleep in an alley next to a local church, receiving food from local restaurateurs. After 2 years of contact, staff noticed she was having difficulty walking. She eventually revealed that her left leg was swollen, but she wasn't worried because she was treating it by wrapping it in kitchen plastic wrap. Two months later, she allowed a team nurse to examine her leg, which was edematous and pale and had numerous areas of purulent fluid beneath the plastic wrap. She refused offers of medical attention because she feared that it would jeopardize her upcoming move into housing, which had been arranged by a church member. After she gave permission to the team, staff shared its medical concerns with the church member, who revealed that Sharon had diabetes. Feeling that this potential risk for sepsis and loss of her limb constituted imminent danger to self, the team brought her involuntarily to an emergency room. She was admitted to the hospital for a course of intravenous antibiotics, her leg was saved, and new housing was achieved. However, she felt a sense of betrayal and refused all further contact with the outreach team.

Sharon's situation illustrates the necessity to be proactive with medical issues. Vigilance alone among all team members can sometimes allow for early identification and sufficient time to educate homeless clients about physical health problems. Her story also highlights the need to be thoughtful about involuntary treatment; such interventions can have both profoundly positive and negative effects, including controversy among team members. In this instance, some staff believed that the decision might have been lifesaving. Others pointed out that although Sharon had survived, she was much less likely to engage with any future care providers. Psychiatrists have a special role regarding involuntary measures, and part of their role as team builders includes encouraging a consensus in treatment planning, while respecting—and learning new strategies from—the views of those who may disagree (McQuistion et al. 2003).

Administrative Issues

Keeping adequate medical records presents special challenges. Clients can refuse to share identifying information, such as their date of birth, their Social Security number, or even their name. Although systems can be created to track clients without such information (e.g., using descriptive nicknames, "dummy" birth dates, or location of contact), they do not suffice for billing purposes. Medical records during the engagement phase primarily serve as a means of transmitting information to other team members.

Another special challenge for medical record keeping involves legal paperwork, such as releases of information and consents for treatment. During engagement, clients are often reluctant to sign any paperwork, although information must be shared with shelters, medical providers, and social service agencies to create unified and complete service plans. Most clients will provide verbal consent for such information exchange; an incentive for housing, for example, is compelling. It is imperative that this verbal consent be documented. A thornier issue exists with consent-for-treatment forms. Clients, especially in the earliest phases of contact, often see the outreach team without formally being "in treatment." In this gray zone the client may accept services from providers without being aware that they are mental health professionals. Nevertheless, all interactions are forms of treatment, and the client's agreement with the interaction implies consent. For this reason, providers ethically should reveal as much as possible about the true nature of their work without sacrificing rapport and trust. Similarly, documenting refusal of contact with the team can rationalize why no treatment was provided.

Legal and Ethical Issues

After a 4-month hospitalization, Mark returned to housing, but not at his previous residence. Unfortunately, to address bureaucratic issues and a change in benefit administration, Mark needed to reapply for entitlements 2 months later. He declined, saying he did not want to sign forms for people he did not know. This eventually led to a termination of SSI and medical coverage, in turn leading to loss of housing and case management services. Mark proceeded to a shelter, where he again refused to sign forms, instead asking shelter staff to talk with the outreach team. He was barred from the shelter because of his refusal to complete appropriate paperwork. The outreach team struggled, and staff discussed whether it could inform shelter personnel of Mark's mental health diagnosis, treatment history, and current reasons for being homeless, all of which could sway the shelter to admit him. However, the team also questioned whether it could share Mark's history of alcohol abuse and nonviolent but objectionable behaviors, which could be equally dissuasive. Mark lived on the streets for 2 weeks until a trusted outreach worker convinced him to sign a release of information between the team and the shelter. The team shared Mark's full history with shelter staff, who agreed to admit Mark if the outreach team visited with him daily and worked to restart medications.

Although it is arguable that verbal consent justifies the exchange of information, outreach teams must still stay within state confidentiality laws and Health Insurance Portability and Accountability Act (HIPAA) guidelines, disclosing only what is necessary. This phase of Mark's experience with the team illustrates how carefully constructed client rapport and thoughtful problem solving among team members resulted in successful referral without violating his rights and compromising his fragile sense of trust. There are no universally correct solutions for these medicolegal issues, and in addition to thoughtful team discussion linked with fastidious chart documentation, teams should also seek collegial consultation, both legal and clinical. These considerations can also be affected by clinician attitudes and countertransference factors. Because of their training, psychiatrists can be particularly valuable as team members in working within the team in this regard (Ng and McQuistion 2004).

From a related ethical standpoint, working with the street homeless presents special challenges. Most prominent is balancing self-determination with paternalism (Melamed et al. 2000). Although a client's decision to participate and succeed in treatment is more likely to be sustained if made self-determinately, making decisions for the client because of safety issues also robs him or her of independence. Is it better to allow clients the freedom to make mistakes, even potentially fatal ones, or to make the "right" decision for the clients "when they are unable" to do so themselves? As in Sharon's case described earlier, each provider must make this decision on an individual case basis.

Safety Issues

Although the goal of any outreach/engagement encounter is to improve the client's condition, safety is paramount. In order to be effective in their work, providers must prioritize the safety concerns of all people involved in the encounter. Public spaces are uncontrolled and present risks of danger to

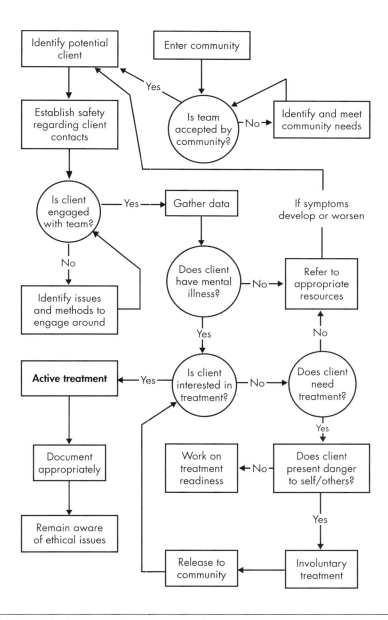

FIGURE 2–1. Flowchart: outreach and engagement.

outreach clinicians and, sometimes, bystanders. Ironically, these risks can derive not only from relatively unknown potential clients but even from passersby themselves (Ng and McQuistion 2004).

Yet approaching homeless people on the street from a rigid structure that "ensures" safety, such as with police, is excessive considering the rarity of physical danger. Moreover, it diminishes rapport and acceptance. A compromise approach involves less structure but emphasizes evasive action when needed. Outreach clinicians should have a low threshold for withdrawing from a clinical encounter until they feel safe engaging the individual. In addition, team members should have set verbal or nonverbal cues to let partners know they have a safety concern. Once a cue is given, team members would have a predetermined plan of how to discuss the concern and what options are available to preserve safety, whether it is disengagement, requesting police backup, or moving to another outreach location.

CONCLUSION

> After 2 weeks in the shelter, Mark agreed to restart medications. A week later, he agreed to sign the necessary paperwork to renew his entitlements. After 2 months of processing, Mark's entitlements were renewed. He reentered case management services and quickly moved into a semi-independent living program. He has remained in this housing program for 5 years, although he is periodically hospitalized for short periods because of continued episodic alcohol use, medication nonadherence, and resultant psychosis.

Engagement of homeless mentally ill individuals often follows a complex path (Figure 2–1), guided by a myriad of unique treatment issues. Only after establishing an accepted presence within the homeless community can the difficult work of engaging disenfranchised individuals begin. As a client's basic needs are met according to his or her own template and timetable, rapport is established. These early experiences will shape not only the client's future treatment, but also his or her motivation to continue in treatment. As engagement progresses, work can begin on obtaining entitlements and addressing the often numerous and advanced medical issues common to this population. Throughout this process, providers must attend to the complex documentation issues, ethical dilemmas, and safety concerns this exciting work often presents.

REFERENCES

Acosta O, Toro PA: Let's ask the homeless people themselves: a needs assessment based on a probability sample of adults. Am J Community Psychol 28:343–366, 2000

Code of Federal Regulations, 24CFR982–985. Washington, DC, U.S. Government Printing Office, April 2005

Desai MM, Rosenheck RA, Kasprow WJ: Determinants of receipt of ambulatory medical care in a national sample of mentally ill homeless veterans. Med Care 41:275–287, 2003

Gelberg L, Linn LS, Usatine RP, et al: Health, homelessness, and poverty: a study of clinic users. Arch Intern Med 150:2325–2330, 1990

McQuistion HL, Felix A, Susser ES: Serving homeless people with mental illness, in Psychiatry, 2nd Edition. Edited by Tasman A, Lieberman J, Kay J. London, Wiley, 2003, pp 2314–2321

Melamed Y, Fromer D, Kemelman Z, et al: Working with mentally ill homeless persons: should we respect their quest for anonymity? J Med Ethics 26:175–178, 2000

Miller WR, Rollnick S, Conforti K: Motivational Interviewing, 2nd Edition: Preparing People for Change. New York, Guilford, 2002

Morse GA, Calsyn RJ, Miller J, et al: Outreach to homeless mentally ill people: conceptual and clinical considerations. Community Ment Health J 32:261–274, 1996

Ng AT, McQuistion HL: Outreach to the homeless: craft, science, and future implications. J Psychiatr Pract 10:95–105, 2004

Nuttbrock L, McQuistion H, Rosenblum A, et al: Broadening perspectives on mobile medical outreach to homeless people. J Health Care Poor Underserved 14:5–16 [erratum: 14(2):290], 2003

Park MJ, Tyrer P, Elsworth E, et al: The measurement of engagement in the homeless mentally ill: the Homeless Engagement and Acceptance Scale–HEAS. Psychol Med 32:855–861, 2002

Prochaska JO, Norcross JC, DiClemente CC: Changing for Good. New York, HarperCollins, 1994

Rowe M, Hoge MA, Fisk D: Services for mentally ill homeless persons: street-level integration. Am J Orthopsychiatry 68:490–496, 1998

Scott J: Homelessness and mental illness. Br J Psychiatry 162:314–324, 1993

Sullivan G, Burnam A, Koegel P, et al: Quality of life of homeless persons with mental illness: results from the course-of-homelessness study. Psychiatr Serv 51:1135–1141, 2000

Waplington J, Morris J, Bradnock G: The dental needs, demands and attitudes of a group of homeless people with mental health problems. Community Dent Health 17:134–137, 2000

Chapter 3

SINGLE ADULTS IN SHELTERS

Elizabeth Oudens, M.D.
Hunter L. McQuistion, M.D.

Michael is a 39-year-old of African American descent who has been in and out of shelters for more than 15 years. He had a chaotic childhood with a history of early maternal loss and physical abuse. He received a diagnosis of schizophrenia in the past and has had multiple psychiatric contacts since age 19, as well as a long history of alcohol, marijuana, and cocaine abuse and several periods of incarceration. He has worked with multiple case managers, several of whom have been frustrated by his frequent relapses, incarcerations, and sporadic availability for services.

UNIQUE ASPECTS OF THE SHELTER SETTING

Individuals staying in shelters are a heterogeneous group, even among those identified as mentally ill. Demographics for homeless adults in the United States indicate that in urban shelters, minorities are overrepresented and men greatly outnumber women (National Coalition for the Homeless 2005). New York City statistics reveal that the majority of individuals staying in shelters are over 40 years old but that there have been an increasing number of young adults ages 18–25 (New York City Department of Homeless Services 2002). Studying shelters in Philadelphia and New York City in the 1990s, Kuhn and Culhane (1998) found that although the "chronically homeless" (those who have been homeless for at least 1 year or four episodes in the past 3 years), made up only 10% of the homeless population over 3 years, they use *half* of all shelter beds on any given night. This group has significantly higher rates of mental illness than the rest of the shelter homeless population, as well as high rates of hospitalization, substance abuse, and medical problems (Kuhn and Culhane 1998).

Generally, mentally ill individuals seen in the shelter system are not able to access community services for several reasons, including denial of illness, inflexibility of traditional health care systems, lack of health insurance, inability to make or follow through with appointments, and mistrust of the system. Many homeless people with mental illness also have had negative experiences of the mental health system. In addition, the homeless population is a vulnerable one. There is evidence suggesting that the experience of a lifetime traumatic event, including childhood physical or sexual abuse, as well as violence experienced while homeless or incarcerated, may be nearly universal among the homeless (Buhrich et al. 2000; Christensen et al. 2005). In our own experience with homeless men, more than 70% report a past traumatic event. Childhood experiences associated with a higher risk of homelessness include a history of foster care or other out-of-home placement, physical or sexual abuse, parental substance abuse, and residential instability and homelessness with one's family as a child (Herman et al. 1997; Koegel et al. 1995). As a result, although individuals seeking shelter have decided to trust enough to come indoors, providing care for psychiatric illness and substance misuse often involves significant outreach and engagement. Providing psychiatric care in the shelter requires taking a long view: the process is a marathon, not a sprint. Although homeless people frequently are thought of as transient, in our experience many return to the same areas or facilities over a period of years. It is important to provide individuals a quality experience of psychiatric service so that even if they are not ready to engage in treatment immediately, they may be willing to accept services in the future.

Homeless shelters in the United States are heterogeneous: small, large; short stay, extended stay; operated in urban and rural areas; run by cities, faith-based organizations, or not-for-profit agencies; serving general or specialized populations. Each has unique services, population, and staffing issues. Funding also varies significantly and can affect the delivery of psychiatric services, including availability of the provider, frequency of contacts, and amount of time spent in direct versus indirect care. Despite these structural and programmatic differences, there are many common aspects of providing psychiatric services in shelters. Several factors set shelter work apart from other types of psychiatric services: 1) services are provided where the person is living; 2) even in the best-run shelters, the nature of shelter life and work is intrinsically chaotic; and 3) psychiatric care is *not* the reason that the person comes to a shelter.

REHABILITATIVE STAGES

Shelter-based care requires a hybrid of emergency room services, street out-reach, and outpatient care. Flexibility is indispensable. The psychiatric provider needs to be skilled in screening, triage, engagement, and collaboration and is typically involved through the stages of the individual's entry into longer-term recovery. McQuistion and colleagues (2003) have described a process of three overlapping stages of rehabilitation for mentally ill homeless people, constituting *engagement* and *intensive care* and culminating in *ongoing rehabilitation*, the stage marked by a person's evolving ability to engage in wellness and recovery, with housing stability, the pursuit of vocational or educational goals, and reestablishment of social ties. Figure 3–1 schematically describes these three stages and the rehabilitative interventions commonly associated with each one of them. The remainder of this chapter focuses on these rehabilitative stages, using Michael's situation as illustration.

Engagement

Owing to incarceration, hospitalization, and brief stays with family members, Michael came in and out of the municipal shelter system over a period of years. Over this time, he worked with a series of case managers. Initially he did not want to meet with a psychiatrist, but he had a relationship with the recreation specialist and some of the longtime shelter staff. The staff would communicate with the psychiatrist and case manager about his condition as soon as he came back to the shelter. Sometimes he needed immediate attention because of the staff's concerns about his weight, his bizarre movements, or his laughing to himself. Although staff initially attributed his behaviors solely to drug use or "acting out," over time they also recognized the symptoms of his mental illness.

Collaborating With the Staff as a Key to Engagement

Effective work in a shelter environment requires a multidisciplinary effort that includes direct shelter staff, case managers, psychiatric provider, and others (e.g., housing specialist, substance abuse counselor, vocational counselor, recreation therapist, medical staff). A psychiatric provider has the best chance of reaching and helping homeless individuals if he or she first builds a relationship with shelter staff colleagues. Although the psychiatric clinician may have the most formal training, it is crucial to recognize that many shelter workers have unsurpassed experience and excellent judgment, intuition, and the ability to form a therapeutic alliance. They have the greatest contact with residents and can often provide a wealth of information about the residents' functioning. In turn, the psychiatric provider can train all shelter staff to help them understand behavioral features of mental illness, such as social with-

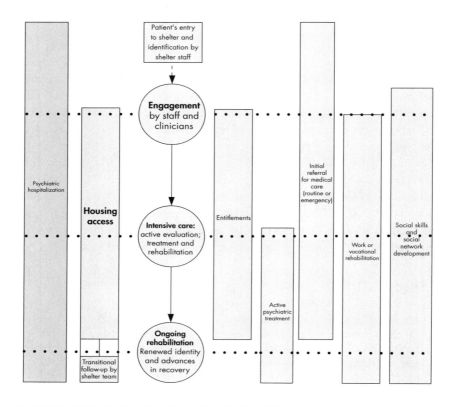

FIGURE 3–1.   Flowchart: stages of rehabilitation.

Circles (with demarcating dotted lines) represent the patient's process through the three stages of rehabilitation. Bars show where key interventions are introduced within these overlapping stages. Access to housing is the cornerstone intervention. Hospitalization is a tool that in some cases aids rehabilitation during all the stages.

drawal, paranoia, or hoarding. However, the level of information needed by line staff differs from that needed by case managers or other clinical staff. While it is essential for the psychiatric provider to solicit input from staff and to educate staff about general psychiatric conditions and associated behaviors, discussing any specific patient information requires consideration of patient confidentiality.

- *Identifying individuals who need assessment.* The psychiatric clinician must be proactive in helping paraprofessional staff recognize behaviors as symptoms by creating ongoing communication with them and educating them to be specific in reporting problematic behaviors. Once an individual has been seen by the psychiatrist, it is important to communicate information back to shelter staff to reinforce the referral, to help them manage behaviors, and to enlist treatment planning ideas.

- *Availability to staff.* It is especially important to be approachable and available to staff. Being visible and friendly, stopping to chat with line staff, attending meetings or spending time out of the consultation room when not seeing patients, and getting involved in crisis situations breaks down some staff members' preconceived notions of a rarefied and remote medical world. This enables staff to seek consultation more freely about engagement and crisis intervention and to learn about mental illness.

Engaging the Individual

> Michael was willing to meet with the psychiatrist and case manager from early on. He enjoyed spending time with others but did not see that he needed attention for mental illness. He was actively using drugs and not consistently available to staff. The clinical staff became used to his not appearing most of the time, set appointments with this assumption, and therefore were late or unavailable when Michael actually appeared. This reinforced his sporadic attendance, requiring the team to make a conscious effort to be consistent in meeting with him. Brief daily visits helped, focusing at first on the day's events and difficulties and only later focusing on his psychiatric condition. It took a number of years before Michael acknowledged his mental illness and addiction. However, by his final year in the shelter, he kept regular weekly appointments with his psychiatrist and case manager.

Good general psychiatric skills serve as a foundation, but some points specific to engaging and treating sheltered homeless individuals deserve special attention.

1. *Be patient.* As is true with the street homeless, the process of engagement is often lengthy and may require outreach over months to years. Many people in shelters have a long history of experiences causing them to mistrust systems, social services, and psychiatric providers.
2. *Be safe.* As in any setting, it is necessary to consider personal safety. Many individuals seen in a shelter may be relatively unknown to staff. Frequently people are intoxicated. In such cases, consider the location and conditions of the interview. The space must afford privacy but cannot be remote. Be sure to have someone else nearby or in the room. In our experience problems are rare, but as in any setting, it is necessary to tune in to your instincts and not ignore warning signs.
3. *Be real.* Sheltered homeless people often are reluctant to meet formally with a psychiatrist. It is important that the prospective patient view the psychiatric clinician as a real object (Susser et al. 1996). Possible approaches include a) asking the staff person who has the most rapport with

the individual to introduce the idea of visiting with a psychiatrist and/or introduce the provider, b) meeting with the person together with someone he or she trusts, c) initiating contact outside of the consultation room, such as sharing coffee in the dining area, playing cards, or taking a walk, and d) keeping initial meetings short.

4. *Be proactive.* Initial contacts may necessitate that the clinician persistently seek out the person. Because the shelter is a living environment, early mornings, dinner, and bed sign-in are productive moments for resident availability. However, it is important to balance a respect for privacy with the need for contact.

5. *Start where the patient is.* This is very important in gaining the individual's participation and trust. Implied in this guideline is approaching each person with respect and hope. What does the individual want? Psychiatric services are often low on the list of the individual's priorities; so on initial contact do not prematurely enter into a mental health history. Similarly, it may not be possible to initiate an ideal treatment plan immediately. Discuss current concerns and how the individual is doing in the shelter: what he or she feels must be accomplished—often housing, work, or a relationship.

6. *Be direct and straightforward.* Sometimes thoughtful self-disclosure is helpful with this population.

7. *Be flexible.* It is not realistic to expect most individuals to show up at appointed times. This is often the goal rather than the starting point and an indicator that can be monitored as treatment progresses.

8. *Be reliable.* It is important to follow through with set appointment times. Not doing so discourages residents from appearing on time, or at all. People in shelters have had experiences queuing up at bureaucracies, in emergency rooms, and in jail or prison, which can evoke feelings of disrespect and lack of control. A sense of reliability and object constancy can also be cultured through scheduling a regular daily or weekly time with a person, even for a few minutes.

9. *Avoid power struggles.* Negotiate. Acceptance and flexibility are required in working with this disaffiliated population.

Intensive Care

Michael presented a complex clinical picture. He had experienced abuse and a number of early losses. He came to the shelter from jail with a diagnosis of schizophrenia but was also chronically using marijuana, crack cocaine, and alcohol. Over the years we got to know more about him by talking with his family members, obtaining old hospital records, speaking with treatment providers during periods of hospitalization and incarceration, and following and evaluating him both during sobriety and relapse. We had the input of all shelter staff, whether they were night staff, recreational workers, or kitchen staff (Michael was in a work stipend program). We saw changes in his mental status after visits with certain family members and on the anniversary of his mother's death, and we learned, together with him, his triggers for stress, relapse, and illness exacerbation. From all of this, we confirmed a diagnosis of schizophrenia, with positive symptoms that markedly worsened when he was using drugs. In addition, as his recovery advanced, feelings of loneliness emerged as well as multiple themes of grief and loss, including the death of his mother, loss of functioning, and lost time.

Homeless individuals present clinical pictures influenced by multiple comorbidities, including substance abuse, trauma, learning disabilities, medical illnesses, and the impact of poverty and living on the streets or in shelters. The following issues are especially relevant to making the diagnosis in a shelter.

Making the Diagnosis

1. *Initial contacts as a series of brief meetings:* These informal contacts serve to engage the patient and formulate an initial impression that is amplified by staff reports.
2. *Advantages of doing assessment in a shelter:* Working where people live provides a unique view of their functioning. It affords the psychiatric provider access to much information, including 24/7 observations by shelter staff, how the individual keeps his or her locker or living space, and how the individual spends his or her time and money. This augments interviews and traditional sources of information such as hospital records or family members.
3. *Understanding personal homelessness history:* A person's trajectory to homelessness episodes typically describes a great deal about functioning, onset and course of illness, and personal vulnerabilities and strengths.
4. *Reassessing diagnoses:* Many arrive with diagnoses from prison, other shelters, or hospitals. Given high rates of comorbidity, diagnostic challenges in this population, and a tendency of systems to pathologize problematic behaviors, it is important to carefully evaluate preexisting diagnoses.
5. *Identifying the timing of symptoms:* To improve diagnostic clarity, it is important to identify the relationship of symptom emergence with substance use, incarceration, and homelessness itself.
6. *Immediate stressors:* Multiple stressors related to homelessness and shelter living exacerbate mental illness, such as lack of money, debt, theft, drug use, fear, uncertain housing, and changes in staff.
7. *Symptoms related to homelessness:* Homelessness itself may create fear, wariness, and a sense of demoralization, independent of diagnosis.

Treatment

Once Michael was staying at the shelter more consistently, we were able to address treatment. He had been prescribed antipsychotic medication in multiple settings: hospital, jail, and the shelter. Although not particularly objecting to medications, he did not see their relevance and took them sporadically. As he became more attached to staff, we arranged a regular morning meeting of 5 to 10 minutes. These visits were coordinated with his medication time so that he took his daily medications, then talked with the psychiatrist. Through this process, we introduced supportive psychotherapy and very concrete, problem-oriented assistance. Each week the case manager prepared a summary of his medication adherence and left him a note at the shelter congratulating or encouraging him. We gave him a pocket-sized calendar and helped him enter phone numbers and appointments. When we introduced regular urine toxicology, Michael chose a start date and was able to accept the intervention as supporting his interest in recovery. He began to attend in-house sobriety groups.

Treatment typically combines medication, supportive psychotherapy, and substance misuse treatment in close coordination with social services. The following points are relevant to integrated treatment:

1. *Treatment planning:* Planning should include specific goals relevant to the individual and to shelter staff. It is important to discuss expectations with the patient and to enlist staff to be alert for changes.
2. *Medication:* It may take a long time for people to accept medication, and prematurely introducing it can hinder the treatment relationship. Even without medication, patients may accept verbal therapies and behavioral approaches. Some considerations when providing medication in the shelter include the following:
   - *Selection for medication therapy:* Consider how likely it is that the person will be available for follow-up. Respect his or her prior experience with medications, including side effects.
   - *Adherence:* Given multiple demands on individuals, simple regimens are preferable. Some people have cognitive deficits or limited experience in organizing and planning appointments. They may benefit from concrete reminders or aids such as calendars, alarm watches and memory books, pillboxes, and blister packs. It is important to account for literacy level when employing some of these aids. Some shelters are able to offer medication monitoring. Incentives for improved adherence relevant to one's own personal priorities are helpful. Depot medication is indicated for those who have a history of poor adherence and who are likely to be available for follow-up.
   - *Safe storage:* Even in a safe, well-run shelter, medications may be misused or stolen for abuse or sale. Possibilities to improve safe storage in-

clude individual lockers or a medication storage/dispensing area if there is staff available to manage it.

- *Access:* Providing access to a full range of medications requires making use of samples and patient assistance programs, as well as familiarity with insurance coverage, especially Medicaid and Medicare Part D.

3. *Substance misuse treatment:* Multiple prevalence studies reveal that substance abuse or dependence is a factor for a large percentage of homeless individuals, including those with a chronic mental illness (Koegel et al. 1999; McCarty et al. 1991; O'Toole et al. 2004). Integrated substance and alcohol treatment is necessary for overall recovery and is preferably managed by the same providers as the mental health treatment.

4. *Hospitalization/crises:* Hospitalization may be necessary, and in our experience, it has been an opportunity to introduce treatment with a person who has not been able to engage with rehabilitation and reaches a point of imminent danger to self or others. It is important to develop clear protocols and to train shelter staff regarding when to call emergency services. Such education also decreases magical expectations regarding hospitalization and its use as a threat or punishment for "bad" behavior. Once a patient is in an emergency room, the psychiatric provider must communicate with emergency department and inpatient staff to provide collateral information and to advocate for the treatment approaches most appropriate to the patient's living circumstances.

5. *Community resources:* These include, but are not limited to, mobile crisis interventions, homeless outreach teams, outpatient treatment programs, clubhouses, vocational programs, and entitlement systems. Familiarity with these services extends homeless people's network while also helping the psychiatric provider engage the patient.

6. *Outside treatment:* Not all psychiatric treatment must take place in the shelter. Some individuals may already be engaged in treatment in the community or be capable of managing it. The shelter team can support this treatment through reminders, coordination with outside services, and possibly role-play of clinic situations, such as asking questions or reporting side effects, to help individuals effectively use traditional services.

Medical Record Keeping and Legal Issues

People frequently cycle in and out of the system, and information is often difficult to access, so good documentation is extremely important. Documentation regarding the path to and length of homelessness, past treatment, medication trials, and response in the shelter, as well as attention to dangerousness, are important elements of the clinical record. As in any setting, the person's consent is required before disclosing personal health information. It can also be helpful to let individuals know how the data is used and to review

with them any specific information being provided for Social Security, rehabilitation, medical treatment, housing, and welfare programs.

Other Health Needs

> Michael was relatively young and healthy, although he did have asthma and
> poor dentition, having lost most of his front teeth. He needed periodic medi-
> cal attention for his asthma and for the dehydration and poor nutrition asso-
> ciated with drug use. These were addressed by a co-located primary care
> clinic, which was able to see him on a drop-in basis until he could follow
> through with appointments. As Michael stabilized on antipsychotic medica-
> tion and maintained sobriety he experienced weight gain, and the medical
> provider worked closely with Michael and his psychiatrist to monitor weight,
> lab tests, and nutrition. Once stable and clean and sober, he was able to ad-
> dress dental care, significantly improving his self-esteem.

In some settings, the psychiatric provider may be the only medical professional an individual sees, requiring the provider to screen for medical conditions, assist in follow-up, and advocate with shelter staff to get health
concerns met. Dental care and lack of access to dental services is also a major
problem for homeless individuals. (Bolden and Kaste 1995; King and Gibson
2003). Collaboration with medical and dental providers who are experienced
and competent in treating mentally ill homeless individuals is essential; shelter co-location of mental health and medical and dental services is ideal. Such
services may be on-site or mobile (Nuttbrock et al. 2003; Project Renewal,
Inc., 2005).

Entitlements

> Michael initially came to the shelter from jail and had neither benefits nor
> prior experience in budgeting. Shelter staff immediately helped him with the
> process of obtaining Medicaid and Social Security benefits. While he was us-
> ing substances heavily the team made the decision to request representative
> payeeship, beginning a money management program with his case manager.
> After Michael had been sober for a year, the psychiatrist provided documen-
> tation to allow him to become his own payee. He continued to learn budgeting
> skills with the support of his case manager.

Individuals are frequently stuck in a demoralizing cycle of multiple in-
complete benefits applications. Work on benefits should start as soon as a person enters the shelter. Medical benefits are essential to providing psychiatric
care, especially medication, and to accessing medical and dental care. The
psychiatric clinician may need to advocate for benefits or identify individuals
who may qualify for psychiatric or physical disability. The provider also
needs to be skilled in building a case for Supplemental Security Income.

When completing a psychiatric evaluation for disability, the clinician should include a clear, specific description of the individual's condition; the impact of symptoms on functioning; and details of medications, including those that potentially affect work function. Providing this information does require the consent of the individual. It is helpful to discuss the application and determination process in advance, and to review specifics of the information being submitted (Drukteinis 2004; Leo and Del Regno 2001).

Housing, Vocational Interests, and Social Connections

> Michael's first job was in the shelter's on-site stipend program. Just before moving out of the shelter, he enrolled in a general equivalency degree (GED) course. As he became clean and sober and entered active psychiatric treatment, Michael spent a greater amount of time with family. His family sought assistance from shelter staff in helping him understand that although they supported Michael, he could not live with them. After years of living in shelters, he had a lot of ambivalence about housing. He was frustrated and impatient with the housing process, and at the same time felt "pushed out" and anxious about living on his own for the first time.

Although not typically the domain of psychiatrists, housing is obviously critical for a shelter-based population. Therefore it is necessary for psychiatrists working in shelters to 1) educate themselves about local housing options and advocate for appropriate housing for their patients; 2) help assess level of functioning with special attention to physical or mental health needs, such as ambulation, medical support, and need for medication monitoring; and 3) provide evaluations for housing placements. In addition, the psychiatrist may need to help the patient adjust to the idea of independent living. Some individuals may have unrealistic expectations about housing. Those who have been homeless for long periods may not perceive supportive housing as desirable because there are greater associated costs, responsibilities, and rules, and therefore they may need help in thinking about a gradual increase in independence. It is important to start with understanding the meaning of housing for the individual.

Some individuals may seek a job or schooling before or in tandem with housing efforts. These goals can provide incentives for sobriety and treatment adherence. Employment or school has multiple benefits, including structure, improved self-esteem, and opportunity for community integration. The psychiatrist can help the individual evaluate these goals and the steps for achieving them. Once the person is employed, it is helpful to foster communication with the clinician and team concerning how the job is going and to ensure that someone is working with the individual to monitor income in relation to disability benefits so as not to jeopardize this safety net. Supported employment programs typically fulfill this need. Although supported employment has not been specifically studied among the homeless mentally ill, studies have clearly shown that the effectiveness of supported employment is generalizable across a range of settings and client characteristics (Bond et al. 2001). Given that homeless individuals who are mentally ill are doubly stigmatized and may have even greater limitations to obtaining employment, they especially need access to programs that support their vocational efforts.

Because of the solitary lifestyle of many single homeless adults with mental illness and/or chemical dependency, their social ties, particularly with family, can be overlooked. For example, in one of our shelters for single men we had a chicken pox outbreak. In the majority of cases, we understood that the men were not in contact with family members. However, as we implemented a municipal Department of Health protocol, men flocked to the phones to call their mothers to see if they had had the virus as children. A knowledge of family relationships can help in understanding the individual's transferential behavior to the shelter team (Fisk et al. 2000). Furthermore, many homeless men and women staying in adult shelters are also parents. It is important to understand and discuss with them the status of their parental rights, relationships with children, and future hopes in relation to their children. In other instances, families do not know the whereabouts of their mentally ill relative and are eager to have contact. Family members can potentially be an important source of information and may help support psychiatric treatment. They may also require considerable psychoeducation. The psychiatric clinician is especially well poised to do this, and thereby supports the social services team in engaging the patient's social network.

Ongoing Rehabilitation: Beyond the Shelter

As formerly homeless individuals enter housing, they begin to acquire a renewed identity that gradually supplants the demoralization of homelessness, advancing their own recovery goals in work and social connection. To optimize this outcome, it is critical to identify good community follow-up before an individual's move to housing. Without sufficient attention to transition, symptoms can be exacerbated and jeopardize success. Transition to housing, while often greatly anticipated, is stressful, especially for those who have been homeless for a long time. One approach shown to significantly decrease subsequent homeless time is Critical Time Intervention (CTI; Susser et al. 1997), designed to provide additional support during the crucial transition period from homelessness to housing. CTI is discussed in detail in Chapter 4 (Psychiatric Emergency Services). Some patients may need to continue with transitional psychiatric care at the shelter while community follow-up is being introduced. The psychiatric provider and the rest of the shelter staff can become very important to the former resident. Although some individuals will want no further contact with the shelter, others need to know that they can return to receive support or to show their progress.

> By the time Michael was ready to leave the shelter, he was keeping weekly meetings with his case manager and psychiatrist. After moving, he was told he could return for these appointments, though his formal psychiatric services were transferred. He was able to use these transitional meetings to support the gains he had made. Michael continues to come by the shelter periodically to let the staff know how he is doing, to show his GED workbooks, and to talk about his new kitten and his job applications. Given his 10-year relationship with the shelter and staff, and the history of loss in his family, this ongoing relationship and ability to touch base has been meaningful. He has now been in the community for a year, engaged in treatment, attending a GED class, visiting with his family, and planning the future.

REFERENCES

Bolden AJ, Kaste LM: Considerations in establishing a dental program for the homeless. J Public Health Dent 55:28–33, 1995

Bond GR, Becker DR, Drake RE, et al: Implementing supported employment as an evidence-based practice. Psychiatr Serv 52:313–322, 2001

Buhrich N, Hodder T, Teesson M: Lifetime prevalence of trauma among homeless people in Sydney. Aust N Z J Psychiatry 34:963–966, 2000

Christensen RC, Hodgkins CC, Garces LK, et al: Homeless, mentally ill and addicted: the need for abuse and trauma services. J Health Care Poor Underserved 16:615–622, 2005

Drukteinis AM: Disability, in The American Psychiatric Publishing Textbook of Forensic Psychiatry: The Clinician's Guide. Edited by Simon RI, Gold LH. Washington, DC, American Psychiatric Publishing, 2004, pp 287–301

Fisk D, Rowe M, Laub D, et al: Homeless persons with mental illness and their families: emerging issues from clinical work. Families in Society 81:351–359, 2000

Herman DB, Susser ES, Struening EL, et al: Adverse childhood experiences: are they risk factors for adult homelessness? Am J Public Health 87:249–255, 1997

King TB, Gibson G: Oral health needs and access to dental care of homeless adults in the United States: a review. Spec Care Dentist 23:143–147, 2003

Koegel P, Melamid E, Burnam A: Childhood risk factors for homelessness among homeless adults. Am J Public Health 85:1642–1649, 1995

Koegel P, Sullivan G, Burnam A, et al: Utilization of mental health and substance abuse services among homeless adults in Los Angeles. Med Care 37:306–317, 1999

Kuhn R, Culhane DP: Applying cluster analysis to test a typology of homelessness by pattern of shelter utilization: results from the analysis of administrative data. Am J Community Psychol 26:207–232, 1998

Leo RJ, Del Regno P: Social Security claims of psychiatric disability: elements of case adjudication and the role of primary care physicians. Prim Care Companion J Clin Psychiatry 3:255–262, 2001

McCarty D, Argeriou M, Huebner RB, et al: Alcoholism, drug abuse, and the homeless. Am Psychol 46:1139–1148, 1991

McQuistion HL, Felix A, Susser ES: Serving homeless people with mental illness, in Psychiatry, 2nd Edition. Edited by Tasman A, Lieberman J, Kay J. London, Wiley, 2003, pp 2314–2321

National Coalition for the Homeless: Who is Homeless? (fact sheet). Updated September 2005. Available at: http://www.nationalhomeless.org/publications/facts/Whois.pdf. Accessed May 2006.

Nuttbrock L, McQuistion H, Rosenblum A, et al: Broadening perspectives on mobile medical outreach to homeless people. J Health Care Poor Underserved 14:5–16 [erratum: 14(2):290], 2003

NYC Department of Homeless Services: Emerging Trends in Client Demographics: Policy and Planning. 2002. http://www.nyc.gov/html/dhs/html/statistics/statistics.shtml. Accessed December 17, 2005.

O'Toole TP, Gibbon JL, Hanusa BH, et al: Self-reported changes in drug and alcohol use after becoming homeless. Am J Public Health 94:830–835, 2004

Project Renewal, Inc: Mobile Medical Outreach Clinic. Available at: http://www.projectrenewal.org/healthcare.html. Accessed December 30, 2005.

Susser ES, Valencia E, McQuistion HL: Critical time points in the care of homeless mentally ill people, in Practicing Psychiatry in the Community: A Manual. Edited by Vaccaro, JV, Clark, GH. Washington, DC, American Psychiatric Press, 1996, pp 259–274

Susser E, Valencia E, Conover S, et al: Preventing recurrent homelessness among mentally ill men: a "critical time" intervention after discharge from a shelter. Am J Public Health 87:256–262, 1997

Chapter 4

FAMILIES IN SHELTERS

Alan Felix, M.D.
Judith Samuels, Ph.D.

Ms. P is a 26-year-old single African American mother of four who entered the shelter to escape an abusive boyfriend. She and her children, ages 1, 4, 7, and 8, were placed into a cramped room in a former motel now being used to shelter homeless families.

Born to parents who were heavily addicted to drugs, Ms. P was neglected and physically abused early in her life. At a young age, she was placed in foster care. Both parents subsequently became infected with HIV, which ultimately claimed the father's life when Ms. P was still a child. Over the course of a number of placements into group and foster homes, she then experienced physical and sexual abuse.

When initially assessed, Ms. P concealed the extent of the domestic violence she and her children experienced prior to the episode of homelessness. She later acknowledged that she did this because she was ashamed and she feared that her children would be taken away from her.

She was able to reveal these important pieces of her family's history only after developing a relationship with her case manager from Family Critical Time Intervention (FCTI), a program designed to facilitate the transition from the shelter into community-based housing and services.

We will describe FCTI later in this chapter as we return to this case to discuss how processes of engagement, case management, and treatment unfolded.

BACKGROUND AND EPIDEMIOLOGY OF HOMELESS FAMILIES

Although research suggests that mental health and substance abuse issues may be common for homeless persons, more recent work suggests that they are probably *not* the reason families are homeless (Rog et al. 1995; Shinn et al. 1998). For example, substance abuse has been found to be a only a small predictor of seeking shelter, and mental illness and substance abuse contribute little to residential instability among poor families (Shinn et al. 1998). It has also been shown that homeless families can probably live outside of "service-intense" environments (Rog et al. 1995) and do as well as poor but not homeless families.

Women in homeless families are younger and are more likely to be from minority groups, to be pregnant or to have recently given birth, and to have lower income and fewer entitlements than women in housed, poor families (Bassuk et al. 1996; Shinn and Weitzman 1996; Shinn et al. 1998). Mothers in homeless families tend to be poorly educated (Shinn et al. 1998) and to have high rates of separation from their families as children, including high rates of placement in foster care (Bassuk et al. 1996).

Risk factors associated with homelessness for families include abuse and separation from the original family in childhood, domestic violence in adulthood, mental health hospitalization in the last 2 years, and abuse of alcohol or heroin (Bassuk et al. 1996; Shinn et al. 1998).

Homeless mothers had a very high lifetime prevalence (72%) of any DSM-III-R disorder as reported by Bassuk et al. in 1996. Lifetime prevalence estimates for specific disorders are 45% for major depressive disorders, 36% for posttraumatic stress disorder (PTSD), and 41% for alcohol/drug abuse. Current prevalence rates are, of course, lower, but still, more than one-third of homeless mothers had a current DSM-III-R disorder in the 1996 study. High prevalence was found for major depressive disorder (10%), PTSD (17%), and alcohol or drug abuse (5%). Almost one-third of the mothers in the study had attempted suicide, and a high proportion had been hospitalized for mental health reasons (12%) or for substance abuse (19%).

Children in homeless family shelters have worse problems with health, mental health, behavior, and educational outcomes than middle-class children, and often than other poor children as well (Rafferty and Shinn 1991; Shinn and Weitzman 1996). Children's internalizing problems such as anxiety and depression have been found to be related to homelessness, and the problems increase with duration, peaking at 3 to 4 months of homelessness (Buckner et al. 1999).

MAKING A DIAGNOSIS: FAMILY ASSESSMENT

A client-centered, empathic, nonjudgmental approach is the key to engagement, which necessarily precedes a clinical assessment. The first meeting with a homeless family should be geared toward clarifying the parents' (usually the single mother's) concerns and priorities. Performing a diagnostic evaluation or initiating psychiatric treatment is a secondary aim and is initiated only when the mother indicates readiness (psychiatric emergencies and crises being the exception). Therefore, the initial history centers on the family's psychosocial history and the events leading to homelessness rather than on a search for psychiatric symptoms. For example, a psychiatric clinician who is offering to help obtain entitlements is more likely to engage a weary mother than the psychiatrist who is perceived to lecture on substance abuse or the importance of psychiatric medication.

Because the family is a systemic unit, the clinician must employ a broader conception of making a "diagnosis" when evaluating a homeless family. Once a family becomes homeless, any combination of the areas of need that we cover in this section may hinder progress into stable community living. For this reason, we believe each area should promptly be assessed after a family becomes homeless, and, in keeping with the Critical Time Intervention (CTI) model (Susser et al. 1997), interventions should target those problems and needs of the family that are most closely linked to persistent homelessness.

In this family assessment, attention is given to the stigma a family experiences due to any or all of the following: homelessness, victimization (e.g., domestic violence, child abuse), mental illness, learning disabilities or illiteracy, substance abuse, poverty, or incarceration of a family member.

Furthermore, we believe that an approach for rapid access to housing (sometimes termed "housing first") must be used whenever possible, addressing the family's needs intensively from the position of their having a secure home. In this way, morbidity related to homelessness can be reduced. Nevertheless, many family shelters and social service agencies require progress toward "housing readiness" before housing is provided to families, unnecessarily prolonging homelessness and problems that may result from shelter life. Figure 4–1 illustrates how the process of assessment and treatment might proceed in concert with rapid rehousing.

Intact couples. The assessment of a homeless family headed by a single mother and one headed by an intact couple will be the same in many cases, but each has unique aspects. Obviously, when a couple is intact, the relationship must be evaluated. The following questions should be raised:

- Which parenting skills are present, and which are lacking, in each parent?
- How does the couple interact in front of the children?
- Is there ongoing family violence?
- Do any members have a serious psychiatric disorder?
- Is couples therapy indicated?
- Is family-focused psychoeducation indicated?

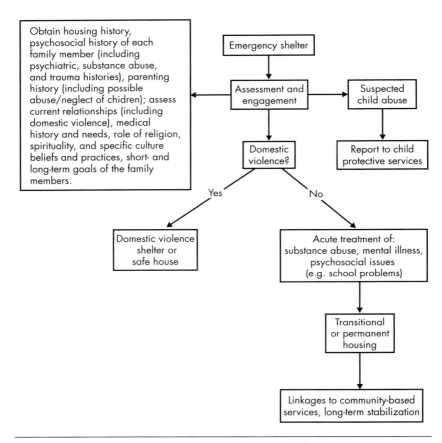

FIGURE 4–1.   Flowchart: assessment of homeless families.

Single parents.   The single-mother household faces its own set of challenges. As with the intact couple, assessment should determine whether or not the mother is in a relationship with a violent partner, whether or not the mother is involved in abuse or neglect of her children, and whether any members have a serious psychiatric disorder. Other questions include the following:

• Is the mother working or capable of working, and if so, how can child care be provided?
• What is the mother's support network?
• Does she need therapy or help with parenting skills?
• Is she attentive to the physical health, mental health, and social, recreational, and educational needs of her children?

It is uncommon for a mother with severe and persistent mental illness to retain custody of her children when she is homeless. Most of the mothers in the FCTI study did not have severe and persistent mental illnesses, but many had histories of depression, personality disorders, trauma-related conditions, and substance abuse disorders. These problems must be carefully assessed by a qualified clinician, often a community psychiatrist. The shelter assessment team or case manager then refers the mother to appropriate treatment services. This may include referral to a domestic violence shelter, outpatient psychotherapy, detoxification or rehabilitation (some such programs, such as modified therapeutic communities, will board the children as well [Sacks et al. 2004]), 12-step programs and other peer support groups, and clinics specializing in trauma therapy.

Family strengths. In the assessment stage of an intervention, several pertinent questions focusing on strengths should be addressed for all family members:

- What is their pattern of relationships with significant people in their lives?
- How motivated are they to change and to accept help?
- To what extent is their identity formed and consolidated, and how much are they capable of advocating for themselves as opposed to depending on others?
- What other psychological strengths do they possess, such as sense of humor, capacity for insight and empathy, or ability to tolerate stress?
- How do they handle anger and disappointment: are they prone to impulsive and violent behavior?

Working as a team. Together with a comprehensive assessment of the family and each member, answers to these questions will usually help the service team know what to expect from the relationship with the family, especially with the head of household.

In this manner, a psychiatrist helps with the determination of the overall service plan beyond the traditional role of diagnostic assessment and treatment. As a clinical supervisor, the psychiatrist may also help direct the case manager to aspects of the family members' histories that are often overlooked. A thorough exploration of the adults' past relationships and experiences, as well as the current family systems dynamics, will help formulate the case management service plan and will also inform the case manager about what to expect as a relationship with the family develops. With ongoing clinical and family systems supervision, this knowledge can be used to prevent or resolve conflicts with and negative reactions toward team members. Likewise, problematic countertransference behavioral responses can be averted.

For example, some mothers encountered in the FCTI study developed the defensive strategy of rejecting help from others because of repeated disappointments in the past. A case manager unfamiliar with this pattern of behavior might withdraw from the client out of frustration. However, one who is knowledgeable about the client's history and sensitive to the psychodynamic meaning of the behavior is less likely to complement the client's maladaptive behavior with her own maladaptive response. Instead, the case manager might offer insight to the client, such as: "You seem to be trying to push me away so that in the end you won't be disappointed, as you have been for so much of your life. I want you to know that no matter how frightened you are of depending on me, and no matter how hard you try to reject my efforts, I will be here to help you when you need me."

UNIQUE ASPECTS OF THE TREATMENT SETTING AND POPULATION

The Treatment Setting

Homeless shelters for families vary throughout the country, but there are three aspects that we believe they all share that differentiate them from permanent housing. Compared with housing, homeless families experience shelters as more dangerous, more stressful, and less private. Out of fear, distrust, shame, and perhaps anger towards the shelter staff, the family may be difficult to engage in the assessment process. Obviously, security must be reliable, and shelter staff should treat the families with respect and dignity.

The lack of privacy in a shelter is a serious concern that should not be overlooked. In the worst scenario, several families share a common room. However, even when families are sheltered in separate living quarters, privacy among family members is typically lacking. This may result in relatively minor concerns, such as a child having trouble finding quiet space to do her homework, or in more serious concerns such as exposing children to adult sexual behavior. Malnutrition-related health problems are also a risk for sheltered families because adequate cooking facilities are rarely available.

Studies of homeless individuals indicate that integrated dual-diagnosis services and interagency cooperation can close service gaps (Rosenheck et al. 2003). Shelter-based interventions for homeless individuals may improve their subsequent treatment engagement in community-based services (Bradford et al. 2005), although Shinn et al. (1998) found that getting services while in a shelter did not predict better outcomes for families and reduced the likelihood of accessing community services such as health care. Also, Rog et al. (1995) found that regardless of the services provided, what made a difference for families was housing. Perhaps these findings reflect the usual problem of lack of continuity of services between shelter settings and housing. Starting and stopping services may be more harmful than not starting them at all. Ideally, shelters would have space on site for comprehensive psychiatric, substance abuse, medical and psychosocial assessment, with continuity of care ensured by a case management team that stayed with the family across the transition into housing. This is the essence of the Family Critical Time Intervention approach described in this chapter. The FCTI approach helps eliminate barriers—whether practical (such as travel costs), psychological (a sense of starting over with strangers), or systemic (lack of coordination between programs or agencies)—to completing the assessment.

The Population and Its Needs

Housing

As we have pointed out, the key intervention with a homeless family is to find adequate housing. There should be enough room to allow for appropriate levels of privacy, ideally in a location preferred by the family. Unfortunately, affordable housing for homeless families is often in the worst neighborhoods, where crime and drug use run high. Nevertheless, stable housing will almost always lower the stress levels within the family and lead to improvement in virtually all areas of need.

Mental Health

The stress of homelessness tends to produce or exacerbate existing psychosocial morbidities. As cited earlier, studies indicate that higher rates of psychiatric disorders occur in homeless adults and children in comparison to domiciled families of similar socioeconomic status. Although depression, PTSD, and substance abuse disorders are often encountered in homeless mothers, symptoms may diminish once suitable housing is found. For example, one study of homeless families in London found that rates of clinically significant psychiatric symptoms decreased from 52% in homeless mothers prior to rehousing to 26% after 1 year during which housing had been obtained (Vostanis et al. 1997). A housing-first approach, where housing is the priority and treatment may then follow, potentially reduces unnecessary utilization of psychiatric services early in the course of homelessness.

The flip side of taking a wait-and-see approach to psychiatric treatment is that the family is likely to have undiagnosed and untreated conditions that could have a negative impact on housing stability, quality of life, and work and school performance. A skilled clinician weighs these different factors and decides when and how to best intervene. A need for individual, group, and family psychotherapies may be inadvertently ignored for homeless families when there are so many practical challenges to their survival. The value of interventions to address psychiatric problems cannot be overstated, and such interventions likely have the added benefit of reducing the risk of future episodes of homelessness.

As described in detail in Drs. Shah and Schacter's chapter on homeless children (Chapter 11), children in homeless families have high rates of psychiatric disorders, learning disabilities, and developmental and behavioral disorders. A comprehensive assessment should include evaluation of developmental delays, sleep problems, eating problems, depression, anxiety, PTSD, aggressive behavior, self-injurious and suicidal behaviors, and psychotic or schizophrenic prodromal signs. When possible, school performance and evaluations should be looked at to assess attentional problems, hyperactivity, and developmental and other learning and behavioral disorders.

Trauma and Domestic Violence

Domestic violence occurs at high rates in this population, and it is often the immediate precipitant of homelessness.

For homeless mothers, victimization is common; 90% report some experience of abuse in their lifetime (Bassuk et al. 1996; Goodman 1991). Incidence of severe partner violence (63%) is also extremely high (Bassuk et al. 1996), nearly three times greater than in the general population (Browne and Bassuk 1997).

The first priority in encountering a homeless family is to determine whether any members are in danger of being harmed. In some cases, an abusive partner will enter the shelter with the family. In other cases, the abuser will track down his victims and continue the abuse. In such cases, placement into domestic-violence shelters is of paramount importance. These shelters vigilantly maintain the anonymity of their residents, carefully blending into their community surroundings to protect the safety of those living there. In addition, they provide peer support groups, counseling, and legal assistance to the victims of violence.

Beyond assessing immediate risk, a community psychiatrist must sensitively obtain the history of violence and trauma in all members of the homeless family. If domestic violence is not an immediate concern, a referral to a peer support group or clinic specializing in domestic violence may suffice. When partners are present, it should not be forgotten that homeless men also have high rates of trauma exposure, most commonly being victims of assault, witnessing death, or experiencing a serious accident or injury. For those with wartime military service, trauma due to combat exposure may be significant. Similarly, even if there is no evidence that children are being abused, it is noteworthy that witnessing domestic violence is traumatic for children and may have a significant impact on their mental health, development, and school performance.

Victims of trauma also are at risk for aggressive behavior. Anger management programs, dialectical behavior therapy, psychopharmacologic interventions, support groups, and other psychotherapies are ways to address the risk of violence in homeless children and adults.

Substance Misuse

Although rates of substance misuse in homeless mothers tend to be lower than those found in homeless single men, there is much at stake for the single mother who experiences this problem. Most notably, she is at risk for losing custody of her children. A nonjudgmental yet thorough history of substance abuse is a necessary part of the assessment. When possible, urine toxicology can be used for the purposes of diagnosis or monitoring. However, these tests must not replace a thorough history and subsequent establishment of open communication with the family on this issue. Savvy users may learn how to get false-negative tests or time their use around expected testing. On the other hand, a single random positive test might lead to unnecessary punitive measures toward a casual user, such as the denial of housing. In other words, it is critical to know people's patterns of use and how they are functionally or symptomatically affected by substance use.

Sobriety is a precondition for subsidized or supportive housing in most social service systems serving homeless families. More progressive programs may house families when the parent or parents have accepted substance abuse treatment, even though abstinence has not yet been achieved. Even more controversial are harm-reduction-based approaches that house families regardless of the stage of recovery, following the theory that stable housing will prevent harm from befalling the family and the chance for recovery will be enhanced.

Motivational interviewing during the initial shelter-based contacts with a family may improve retention in substance abuse treatment programs (Carroll et al. 2006). Twelve-step programs remain a foundation for chemical dependency treatment. "Double-trouble" programs (which address coexisting mental illness and substance abuse), as well as the use of pharmacologic and other somatic interventions such as acupuncture, can enhance 12-step interventions.

Entitlements

A case manager typically is responsible for coordinating applications for entitlements for homeless families. A service team facilitates access to programs such as Temporary Assistance for Needy Families (TANF) and other public assistance, food stamps, Social Security entitlements, Medicaid and Medicare, and Section 8 and other subsidized housing programs.

The community or public sector psychiatrist plays an important role in determining psychiatric or other medical disability and in determining capacity to manage benefits (e.g., determinations of payee status or custodial care). Psychiatrists and other health care providers must give high priority to addressing the family's insurance status so that access to care will not be denied. For the uninsured (those with pending benefit applications and those who are undocumented), access to free clinics, medication grant programs, and sample medications should be considered.

Education

Educational and employment goals are often priorities for homeless mothers. Helping them identify a means to resume their education or helping them resolve academic problems faced by their children is often an excellent way to form a clinical alliance. As noted earlier (and as illustrated below in the second part of Ms. P's case history), a child's problems in school may provide a clue to other problems faced by the homeless family. Likewise, the clinical team's efforts to assess a child's school problems can be coordinated with those of teachers and counselors at the school.

Employment

Homeless mothers, like their housed but impoverished counterparts who receive welfare (TANF), are under increased pressure to find and maintain employment. Assessment of the mother's job skills, interests, and goals will help determine whether additional job training is necessary to enable her to seek competitive employment. Treatment of psychiatric conditions that interfere with employment is critical. For mothers who have a chronic mental illness or who are in recovery from chemical dependency, supportive employment programs may be suitable (Mueser et al. 2004; Salyers et al. 2004).

Medical and Dental

A psychiatrist may be the first person to recognize signs of dental, ophthalmologic, and other medical problems among homeless populations. These are usually poorly attended chronic problems like dental abscesses, caries, glaucoma, diabetes, hypertension, thyroid conditions, hypercholesterolemia, and asthma that may have gone undetected in homeless mothers. Children may not have received adequate immunizations and may suffer from poor nutrition or from lead exposure due to substandard living conditions.

On-site or mobile medical teams (Nuttbrock et al. 2003) able to provide assessment and basic care at intake shelters offer a way to overcome the barriers to health care typically faced by homeless families. (Usatine et al. 1994)

Parenting Skills and Child Care

Most homeless mothers have good or even excellent parenting skills but need extra support when confronted with the crisis of homelessness. Parenting skills classes are especially useful to young first-time mothers. In addition, there is some evidence that parenting education can help reduce abusive behaviors in homeless mothers (Gorzka 1999).

To support parenting and enable mothers to work or resume their educations, access to free or affordable good-quality child care is essential. Case managers may refer families to their own agency's child care services, if available, or help the mother locate a provider.

Record Keeping

A unique challenge faced when working with families is to document family issues in a way that protects the confidentiality of each member. One has to keep in mind that notes kept in the mother's record should not divulge too much detail about the children, a spouse, or a significant other. This presents a challenge to record keepers because many of the mother's concerns may center on the other members of the family, and thus confidential information about a spouse or child could be unwittingly revealed through the release of her record. Furthermore, the mother's record may be released with her consent only. For these reasons, we recommend that separate records be kept for each family member, and/or that separate, more detailed records be made that specifically deal with family issues.

FCTI: A MODEL PROGRAM FOR HOMELESS FAMILIES

The Family Critical Time Intervention program in Westchester County, New York, illustrates the principles and services we have described. FCTI has two components: 1) rapid placement in transitional housing and 2) intensive short-term FCTI case management. Because the housing is considered temporary, one of the primary goals for the families is to work toward permanent housing.

FCTI workers provide motivational support for mothers and assist them in seeking treatment and services by helping with service referrals, linkages, and integration. FCTI workers have comprehensive knowledge of providers in the community that offer appropriate treatment and services for the mother. Although FCTI workers have training specifically related to issues of trauma and case work, they do not directly provide trauma services. Instead, they make referrals to other providers to strengthen family members' long-term ties to services, family, and friends and provide emotional and practical support during the critical time of transition from a shelter to temporary housing and permanent housing. Over a 9-month period, the program has three 3-month phases that can shift and overlap according to client family needs: 1) transition to community, 2) practicing phase, and 3) transfer of care (Susser et al. 1997; Valencia et al. 1997).

Three Phases of Care

The first stage, *transition to community,* begins when the FCTI case manager is introduced to a family shortly after the family arrives at the shelter. The case manager's main role during this phase is to help the mother complete the shelter assessment and begin the key task of linking the mother and family to appropriate community resources.

The *practicing phase* is devoted to testing and adjusting the support systems established while at the shelter and after the family's move into the community (Valencia et al. 1997). The FCTI worker observes where the mother and family need more or fewer supports and services, targeting areas that need more work. The goal during this phase is for the caseworker to allow the mother the space to maximize her strengths while remaining available to help in areas where the mother is having difficulties coping. The task for the worker, then, is to advance trust while providing boundaries regarding dependency as the mother copes with the new changes in her family's lives (Caton et al. 1994; Susser et al. 1991). If possible, the worker begins to step back during this phase and become less active with the family.

During the final phase, *transfer to care,* fine-tuning is done to the support system to ensure that long-term community-based linkages are established (Valencia et al. 1997). Transfer of care means that the family remains in transitional or permanent housing, but the FCTI case manager transfers those services that are still needed to community-based providers and other supports.

Role of the Psychiatrist

Throughout the stages of FCTI, a psychiatrist may play several roles. In the Westchester study, a psychiatrist met with the case management and supervisory social work staff weekly to hear case presentations and to help the team formulate a comprehensive treatment plan. A child psychiatrist was also available to consult on challenging cases involving the children enrolled in the program. In subsequent team meetings, the family was often invited in to meet with the psychiatrist, or the team would go to the family's home once they were placed into housing. In addition to consulting on the overall treatment plan, another important role of the psychiatrist was to assess and address difficult transference/countertransference binds between family members and the case manager. Occasionally, the psychiatrist was asked to advocate for specific services on behalf of the family (e.g., mental health treatments, school-based interventions, benefit applications). Lastly, it was the psychiatrist's role to help ensure fidelity to the CTI model of care, typically by reigning in an overzealous case manager who was having difficulty stepping back toward the end of the intervention.

Overcoming Family Homelessness and the Road to Recovery

The process of assessing Ms. P and her family really began with Ms. P forming an alliance with her CTI case manager with the aim of moving the family into a transitional apartment. Once they were housed, Ms. P sought help for her 8-year-old daughter, who was having trouble in school due to aggressive behavior toward other students. The CTI case manager encouraged Ms. P to bring her daughter to the weekly CTI clinical meeting attended by case managers, social work supervisors, and adult and child psychiatrists.

At the weekly meeting, Ms. P revealed for the first time the full extent of her own childhood abuse, as well as the extensive domestic violence she endured in virtually all of her adult relationships. In discussing her daughter's problems, Ms. P acknowledged that her children frequently witnessed the violent outbursts of her boyfriend, who was now incarcerated. She was currently depressed and had been taking antidepressant medication since the onset of postpartum depression with the birth of her youngest child, although she was only able to see her prescribing internist every 3–4 months. She had also shied away from seeing psychiatrists because she feared she would have to "talk about things too much."

As a result of the conference, Ms. P accepted a referral to a psychiatrist and agreed to have her daughter evaluated as the school was recommending. Ms. P's depression improved with more aggressive treatment, and she was able to obtain a job as an aide in a nursing home. Things were going well until the seventh month of CTI, when the case manager left to take another job. Despite having been prepared for this change, Ms. P reacted to the new case manager by initially refusing to return all calls. When the new case manager showed up at Ms. P's apartment with a letter (in case no one was home), Ms. P assumed it was an eviction notice and became quite angry. This was a rocky start to the final 2 months of CTI, when the important task of obtaining permanent housing still remained. Things were complicated by Ms. P's use of splitting as a defense, idealizing her former case manager who "let me make my own rules" and devaluing the new one.

Another CTI team meeting was held with Ms. P in her own apartment. At that meeting, she revealed how the loss of her case manager reverberated with her past experience of abuse and neglect. Referring to her new case manager, she said, "All she wants to do is bang on me." Through having a chance to talk about how she missed her former case manager and to consider that she was negatively distorting the intentions of her new worker, Ms. P was able to become less angry and more receptive to working on the final task of moving into permanent housing and terminating from CTI. The team praised her for diligently maintaining her apartment, for taking care of her children so well, and for sustaining a job (no easy task for mothers under far better socioeconomic conditions). The meeting ended with Ms. P smiling with tears in her eyes, saying, "I just wanted somebody to give me a pat on the back."

REFERENCES

Bassuk EL, Weinreb LF, Buckner JC, et al: The characteristics and needs of sheltered homeless and low-income housed mothers. JAMA 276:640–646, 1996

Bradford DW, Gaynes BN, Kim MM, et al: Can shelter-based interventions improve treatment engagement in homeless individuals with psychiatric and/or substance misuse disorders? A randomized controlled trial. Med Care 43:763–768, 2005

Browne A, Bassuk S: Intimate violence in the lives of homeless and poor housed women: prevalence and patterns in an ethnically diverse sample. Am J Orthopsychiatry 67:261–278, 1997

Buckner JC, Bassuk EL, Weinreb LF, et al: Homelessness and its relation to the mental health and behavior of low-income school-age children. Dev Psychol 35:246–257, 1999

Carroll KM, Ball SA, Nich C, et al: Motivational interviewing to improve treatment engagement and outcome in individuals seeking treatment for substance abuse: a multisite effectiveness study. Drug Alcohol Depend 81:301–312, 2006

Caton CL, Shrout PE, Eagle PF, et al: Risk factors for homelessness among schizophrenic men: a case-control study. Am J Public Health 84:265–270, 1994

Goodman LA: The prevalence of abuse among homeless poor mothers: a comparison study. Am J Orthopsychiatry 61:489–500, 1991

Gorzka PA: Homeless parents: parenting education to prevent abusive behaviors. J Child Adolesc Psychiatr Nurs 12:101–109, 1999

Mueser KT, Clark RE, Haines M, et al: The Hartford study of supported employment for persons with severe mental illness. J Consult Clin Psychol 72:479–490, 2004

Nuttbrock L, McQuistion HL, Rosenblum A: Broadening perspectives on mobile medical outreach to homeless people. J Health Care Poor Underserved 14:5–16 [erratum: 14(2):290], 2003

Rafferty Y, Shinn M: The impact of homelessness on children. Am Psychol 46:1170–1179, 1991

Rog DJ, McCombs-Thornton KL, Gilbert-Mongelli AM, et al: Implementation of the homeless families program, 2: characteristics, strengths, and needs of participant families. Am J Orthopsychiatry 65:514–528, 1995

Rosenheck RA, Resnick SG, Morrissey JP: Closing service system gaps for homeless clients with a dual diagnosis: integrated teams and interagency cooperation. J Ment Health Policy Econ 6:77–87, 2003

Sacks S, Sacks JY, McKendrick K, et al: Outcomes from a therapeutic community for homeless addicted mothers and their children. Adm Policy Ment Health 31:313–338, 2004

Salyers MP, Becker DR, Drake RE, et al: A ten-year follow-up of a supported employment program. Psychiatr Serv 55:302–308, 2004

Shinn M, Weitzman BC: Homeless families are different, in Homelessness in America. Edited by Baumohl J. Phoenix, AZ, Oryx Press, 1996, pp 109–122

Shinn M, Weitzman BC, Stojanovic D, et al: Predictors of homelessness among families in New York City: from shelter request to housing stability. Am J Public Health 88:1651–1657, 1998

Susser ES, Lin SP, Conover SA, et al: Childhood antecedents of homelessness in psychiatric patients. Am J Psychiatry 148:1026–1030, 1991

Susser E, Valencia E, Conover S, et al: Preventing recurrent homelessness among mentally ill men: a "critical time" intervention after discharge from a shelter. Am J Public Health 87:256–262, 1997

Usatine RP, Gelberg L, Smith MH, et al: Health care for the homeless: a family medicine perspective. Am Fam Physician 49:139–146, 1994

Valencia E, Susser E, Torres J, et al: Critical time intervention for individuals in transition from shelter to community living, in Innovative Programs for the Homeless Mentally Ill. Edited by Breakey WR, Thompson JW. Amsterdam, Harwood Academic, 1997, pp 75–94

Vostanis P, Grattan E, Cumella S, et al: Psychosocial functioning of homeless children. J Am Acad Child Adolesc Psychiatry 36:881–889, 1997

Chapter 5

ASSERTIVE COMMUNITY TREATMENT

Ann Hackman, M.D.
Lisa Dixon, M.D.

ASSERTIVE COMMUNITY TREATMENT: A CASE EXAMPLE

Making a diagnosis. Mr. D was a 34-year-old African American male who had been homeless for more than 10 years when he was identified by outreach workers as someone with a psychiatric illness and was referred to the University of Maryland Assertive Community Treatment (ACT) team in 1993. Mr. D experienced symptoms including auditory hallucinations and paranoid delusions; he was extremely isolated, avoided shelters, slept on the streets, and had difficulty with activities of daily living. Although he had been arrested several times for crimes including loitering and trespassing, he had avoided psychiatric hospitalization and treatment. (In Maryland, the statute regarding involuntary hospitalization required that an individual present a clear and present danger to self or others.) Over a series of visits, a diagnosis of schizophrenia was made based on the patient's clinical presentation.

Access to entitlements. At the time of his admission to ACT, Mr. D was not receiving any entitlements, nor had he ever received any, despite a decade of homelessness. He was assisted in obtaining entitlements (Supplemental Security Income [SSI] and Medicaid) through the SSI Outreach Project, a Substance Abuse and Mental Health Services Administration–funded program that allows presumptive assessment of disability and rapid receipt of funds.

Engagement. When the ACT team initially began to engage Mr. D, he had extremely poor hygiene and self care. Engaging him in treatment occurred over the course of a year, with team members, including his primary therapist, his psychiatrist, and a consumer advocate, meeting him several times a week behind a fast food restaurant. Team members brought Mr. D food, shoes, clothing, and other necessities of daily life. He was encouraged to come into the ACT office to use shower and laundry facilities but was reluctant to do so. Although he accepted food and clothing, he initially refused housing and medication. After several months, as weather grew colder, Mr. D was persuaded to go into housing, and a room was obtained for him in a board and care facility.

Development of a treatment plan. It was only after Mr. D was in housing with some of his basic needs being met that the team was able to move beyond engagement and into active treatment. Challenges at this point included Mr. D's reluctance to bathe and the fact that he had lice. His male psychiatrist assisted him in using the treatment for lice. However, Mr. D continued to refuse to bathe regularly, thus jeopardizing his housing, until team members discovered that Mr. D was willing to take bubble baths and purchased the appropriate products for him. His housing remained at risk because of his disorganization and consequent inability to keep his living space clean and safe; Mr. D had worked with ACT for more than a year before he was persuaded to undergo a trial of depot medication.

On medication he made gradual improvement and became more organized in his thinking, his self-care, and his attention to his living area. He expressed the desire to have his own apartment, and after considerable discussion and preparation (including practicing using a microwave), he was assisted in finding and renting an apartment that he was able to maintain successfully. With minimal assistance from the team, Mr. D obtained a driver's license and purchased a car with SSI money that he had saved. With help from the team's family outreach coordinator, Mr. D reestablished interaction with several family members; he later developed a friendship with another resident in his building.

Ongoing rehabilitation. Mr. D. was transitioned from ACT to traditional community mental health services in the University of Maryland system. He has been able to engage with these services, keeps scheduled appointments, is adherent with medication, and has successfully remained in treatment there for the past 5 years. He maintains occasional contact with ACT staff, sometimes stopping in for a cup of coffee; he reports that he feels things are going well.

KEY ELEMENTS, STRUCTURE, AND FUNCTION OF ACT

All patients who are homeless and have severe mental illness and who receive ACT services do not have the same outcome as Mr. D. However, ACT services can be extremely helpful to homeless people with mental illness. In this chapter we review the ACT model and its origins, consider populations in which the model has been employed, and report on several programs designed specifically to provide ACT services to homeless patients, with specific focus on the Baltimore ACT program with which we have been involved.

ACT began in the early 1970s as the Training in Community Living model at the Mendota Mental Health Institute in Madison, Wisconsin (Marx et al. 1973). Drs. Stein, Test, and Marx developed an innovative approach to treatment in the community of patients with schizophrenia and extensive histories of past hospitalization, entailing both psychiatric treatment and assistance with daily living. Many hospital-like services were provided in a community setting. A randomized controlled study found the approach to be effective in reducing hospitalization and decreasing symptoms while increasing employment and improving social relationships and life satisfaction (Test and Stein 1980); the program was also found to be cost effective (Weisbrod et al. 1980).

ACT has since become widely utilized, and the model has been found to include certain critical elements. Critical components include multidisciplinary staff, team approach, small caseload, high intensity, community locus, assertive engagement, staff continuity, collaboration with support system, and continuous responsibility (McGrew and Bond 1997; McHugo et al. 1999). Fidelity to the model has been emphasized, and research has shown that greater fidelity is associated with better outcomes (McHugo et al. 1999).

In their text on ACT, Stein and Santos (1998) recommended the following regarding the structure, organization, and functioning of ACT teams: A team should range from 8 to 15 employees and have professional and nonprofessional staff, including social workers, psychiatric nurses, and counselors; it should include a psychiatrist and optimally also an addictions counselor, a job coach, and a peer counselor. The team, which should meet daily, shares responsibility for the patients (the entire team getting to know all patients), and the therapist-to-patient ratio should be small (optimally about 1:10). Patients should have individualized treatment plans, receive integrated services, and be seen frequently, as often as several times a day. Much of the service provided should occur in the community (in the patient's home, day program, workplace, or other community settings); patients need to have some access to the team 24 hours a day. The team needs to be assertive in its approach to clients and to the community. At the same time, the team should relate to patients as responsible individuals and capitalize on their strengths. The team should work with the patient and with his or her family (sometimes providing family psychoeducation) and support system (including employers and housing providers) throughout the patient's time with the team; the team should provide continuous care, following patients when they are hospitalized or incarcerated. While not necessarily continuing indefinitely, ACT services are not limited to a predetermined time period and should continue for as long as the patient needs them.

POPULATIONS AND SETTINGS

As noted by Dixon (2000) in a detailed article on the history of ACT, the model has been studied in a variety of populations in settings both rural (Becker et al. 1999; Calsyn et al. 1998) and urban (Dixon et al. 1993; Lehman et al. 1997) and with veterans (Rosenheck and Neale 2004). There have been international applications, including extensive implementation in Canada (Chue et al. 2004), established programs in England (Burns et al. 2001; Priebe et al. 2003), new programs elsewhere in Europe including Poland (Zaluska et al. 2005) and Denmark (Aagaar and Nielsen 2004), as well as ACT teams in Sweden, Germany, and Italy (Burns et al. 2001), and programs elsewhere in the world including Australia (Hambridge and Rosen 1994) and Singapore (Lim et al. 2005). ACT has also been used in the treatment of patients with personality disorders (Tyrer and Simmonds 2003). It has also been tested with a program that employs a combination of ACT with family psychoeducation (McFarlane 1997; McFarlane et al. 1992, 1996). A modified version of ACT has been employed with forensic populations (Lamberti et al. 2004; McCoy et al. 2004). Although the initial Training in Community Living program excluded individuals with co-occurring substance use disorders, it has been found that with minor adjustments, the program can be very effective in treating dually diagnosed individuals (Drake et al. 1998; Meisler et al. 1997; Teague et al. 1995). The ACT approach to treatment is currently a part of most best-practices standards and is included in the Schizophrenia Patients Outcome Research Team (PORT) recommendations (Lehman and Steinwachs 1998; Lehman et al. 2004).

STUDIES OF ACT PROGRAMS AND ELEMENTS

The use of ACT services with homeless individuals was first studied in the early 1990s (Dixon et al. 1995; Lehman et al. 1997; Morse et al. 1992, 1997) and has been evaluated further in programs including Pathways to Housing (Tsemberis and Eisenberg 2000) and Access to Community Care and Effective Services and Supports (ACCESS) (McGuire and Rosenheck 2004; Randolph et al. 2002; Rosenheck and Dennis 2001). This chapter describes other studies but focuses on the work of Lehman and Dixon with the Baltimore ACT team.

Morse and colleagues (1992) compared a continuous treatment team, a drop-in center, and a traditional community mental health center that each provided treatment of homeless individuals with serious mental illness over a 12-month period. They found that although individuals in all three treatment groups showed improvement over baseline measures, patients working with the continuous treatment team had more contact with the program and used more community resources, reported greater satisfaction with the program, and experienced fewer days of homelessness. In further work in an 18-month study of individuals with severe mental illness who were homeless or at risk for homelessness, Morse and colleagues (1997) compared broker case management with traditional ACT alone and with ACT augmented by additional supports from community workers. Patients in both ACT conditions had more contact with their assigned treatment program, better resource utilization, less severity of thought disorder, greater activity levels, and higher scores on client satisfaction measures. Patients receiving traditional ACT alone had more days in stable housing than those in the other two groups. The authors concluded that ACT is superior to broker case management for homeless individuals with severe mental illness.

Pathways to Housing (Tsemberis and Eisenberg 2000) provided supported housing to homeless individuals in combination with somewhat modified ACT services; supported housing involved immediate placement of homeless individuals with severe mental illness in their own apartments chosen from units available on the open market. Consumers were required to meet with staff a minimum of twice a month and to participate in a money management plan; other services, including mental health, somatic, and substance abuse treatment and vocational services, were made available to clients who could determine the type and intensity of services they wanted to receive. This group was compared with homeless individuals with severe mental illness who received housing through traditional channels. After 5 years, 88% of the individuals in the Pathways program remained in housing, whereas only 47% of the comparison group remained housed.

ACCESS was a 5-year multisite demonstration program developed to address fragmented care received by homeless persons with severe mental illness and to evaluate the effect of implementing system change strategies designed to improve interagency collaboration and cooperation (Randolph et al. 2002). Part of the program included the provision of intensive outreach and time-limited ACT services. As described by Rosenheck and Dennis (2001) in their evaluation of outcomes for patients in the fourth annual cohort of ACCESS, the program was designed for patients to receive ACT services for 1 year, although the actual time of discharge was determined by the clinician, with some patients leaving in less than 12 months and others staying for more than 18 months. They compared outcomes in patients who had been discharged at the time of 3-, 12-, and 18-month follow-ups with those who had not been discharged; they found no significant differences between the two groups on measures of mental health, substance abuse, and housing. However, the patients who had been discharged had significantly less health service use (on all measures except hospital days) than those who remained in treatment with the ACT teams; discharged individuals had worked for more days than those still enrolled in the program. Clients with longer duration of treatment had improved outcomes on measures of drug use and housing. Clients who were judged by their case managers to have successfully completed the program (only 3% of the individuals discharged) had better outcomes on all measures. The authors conclude that homeless individuals with severe mental illness benefit from ACT and that they can be selectively discharged and transferred to other services (such as high- or low-intensity case management) without deterioration in mental health, substance abuse, housing, or employment status.

THE BALTIMORE ACT TEAM

The Baltimore ACT team began in 1991 as the experimental arm of a randomized clinical trial designed to assess the efficacy of ACT with homeless adults with mental illness as compared with standard treatment. Patients treated in the ACT program were found to have more psychiatric outpatient visits and fewer hospital days and emergency department visits than comparison subjects; they also spent more days in stable housing and demonstrated improvement on measures of symptoms, life satisfaction, and perceived health status (Lehman et al. 1997). Dixon and colleagues (1995) described some modifications that the Baltimore program made in the ACT model to facilitate the provision of services to homeless individuals with severe mental illness. The team philosophy held that clients' quality of life improves when individuals are engaged in a nonthreatening and nonintrusive manner, are provided help with obtaining housing entitlements and medical care, and are assisted in functioning in the community. ACT treatment was conceptualized in four phases (Dixon et al. 1995). The first was *engagement,* with the goal of developing a trusting relationship between the team and the client. During this phase the team worked in community settings to assist the client with basic needs and maintained the contact, including when a client was hospitalized or arrested; the psychiatrist also maintained regular contact even if the client was not taking or was refusing medications. The second phase was *stabilization,* during which the team assisted the client in developing skills essential to maintaining a stable lifestyle in the community and collaborated with the client in addressing problems including the following: securing long-term housing, obtaining and maintaining regular income, achieving daily structure, treating chronic medical issues, addressing substance use problems, and enhancing family and interpersonal relationships, as well as addressing psychiatric problems. The third phase was *maintenance and ongoing treatment,* during which the client was assisted, often with less intense services than orig-inally required, in maintaining gains and making further progress; steps in this phase might include moving from a psychosocial program to employ-ment or from having a representative payee to managing money indepen-dently. The final phase of treatment with the Baltimore ACT team was *discharge,* which was considered when the client and the team agreed that the client had met the goals of treatment; the discharge process was carefully planned, often taking several months. Clients were transitioned from the ACT team to treatment in less intensive mobile outreach programs, case management programs, and standard clinics.

The ACT model was modified to facilitate the provision of services to a homeless population (Dixon et al. 1995). Some of the changes involved the addition of several staff positions, including outreach workers, consumer ad-vocates, and a family outreach coordinator. Outreach workers were a part of the research protocol and were responsible for identifying prospective pa-tients in the community; patients were recruited from shelters, soup kitchens, and drop-in centers as well as from on the street; the outreach workers were only peripherally involved with day-to-day functions of the team. The team had two consumer advocates; these were individuals with backgrounds of mental illness and/or homelessness who worked closely with clients as advo-cates and peer counselors and sometimes performed some case management services, although not having primary responsibility for a caseload; the con-sumer advocates were extremely important team members and helped to cre-ate a more positive attitude in the team toward people with mental illness (Dixon et al. 1994, 1997). The family outreach coordinator was a part-time position funded through NAMI (now the National Alliance on Mental Ill-ness); most patients had some contact with their families and, in part through the efforts of the family outreach worker, the team was able to establish con-tact with families and to provide some education and support. Work with families was associated with higher levels of satisfaction with family relations and with stable housing (Dixon et al. 1998).

Other changes to the ACT model involved the way in which services were provided and included the utilization of mini-teams made up of a case man-ager, a psychiatrist, and a consumer advocate; the use of drop-in and office-based services; and the assumption of a time-limited framework for treatment (Dixon et al. 1995). The decision to use mini-teams with assigned case manag-ers for each patient rather than the shared caseloads of the original ACT model was made based on the belief that engagement with homeless individuals could best be achieved if the patients were seeing a small number of individuals consistently rather than having outreach from a dozen different people. In ad-dition to providing services in the community, the Baltimore ACT team found that with a homeless population, many individuals were quite willing to come

TREATMENT PLAN: MR. D

<u>Initial</u> (within 45 days of admission)   **Completion Date: 9/30/93**

Client treatment expectations	DSM-IV diagnosis	Referral plans
Client unable to identify any expectations at this time	**Axis I:** Schizophrenia, CUT **Axis II:** Deferred **Axis III:** Unknown **Axis IV:** Homelessness, chronic mental illness, no entitlement **Axis V:** 30	Somatic and dental referrals indicated

Individual strengths	Current medications	Allergies
Ambulatory No known medical problems Survival skills	None	Unknown
		Weight
		Unknown

<u>Long-term goals</u> *(Goals related to presenting problems, symptoms. Specify goal for each problem.)*

Goal target date
1. Patient will be engaged in treatment with ACT team and will identify team as his treatment provider: 9/30/94
2. Patient will accept medications and other treatment for his psychiatric symptoms: 9/30/94
3. Patient will allow physical examination: 3/30/94
4. Patient will obtain and maintain safe and appropriate housing: 3/30/94
5. Patient will receive SSI and medical entitlements: 3/30/94
6. Patient will be transitioned to less intensive services: 9/30/96

<u>Progress on objectives</u> *(Describe progress on each short-term goal of previous ITP.)*

N/A

<u>Problem list/short-term objectives</u>

Problems/symptoms	Short-term objectives	Intervention modality	Staff	Frequency	Target date
1. Engagement	Patient will be available to meet with ACT staff 2x/week	Outreach	Ms V, LCSW; Dr. R, PGY-IV; Dr. D; Ms. M; CA	Visits 3–4x/week	12/30/94
2. Psychiatric illness as evidenced by auditory hallucinations, paranoia, poor self-care	Deferred				
3. Unknown medical status	Deferred				
4. Homelessness	Deferred				
5. Lack of entitlements	Deferred				

Signatures: Ms. V, LCSW; Dr. R., PGY-IV resident; Dr. D, attending psychiatrist; Ms. M.; consumer advocate; other team members

FIGURE 5–1.   Individual treatment plan for Mr. D.
ACT=Assertive Community Treatment; CUT=chronic undifferentiated type; SSI= Supplemental Security Income.

into the office, where in addition to other services there were facilities available for meals, bathing, and laundry. The team provided coffee for patients in the mornings and offered some groups. Many patients had difficulty keeping specific appointments but were able, for example, to come in on a designated afternoon or day of the week. Encouraging patients to come into the office

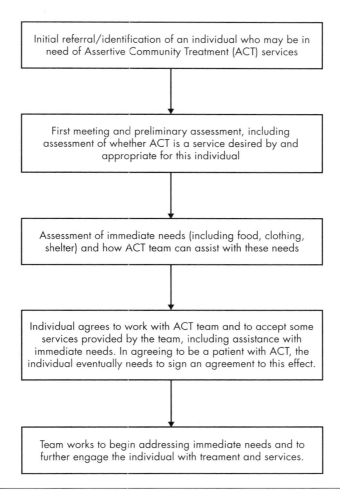

FIGURE 5–2. Flowchart: initial engagement phase of Assertive Community Treatment.

allowed the entire staff to get to know all the patients and facilitated the process of preparing individuals for transition to less intensive services. Although there was not a specific time limit on services, patients were evaluated annually for readiness to make the transition. In working with a population of homeless patients there were many individuals who had experienced few hospitalizations, had little understanding of their illnesses, and had limited experience with outpatient care. Once such patients had obtained housing, addressed other needs, and learned to successfully manage their illnesses, they were often able to move to less intensive services; patients typically saw this as a graduation and were proud of being able to take increased responsibility for their lives.

The Baltimore ACT team has continued its operations with several further modifications. The team currently (2005) serves domiciled as well as homeless individuals, although a majority of patients continue to have histories of homelessness. Services are reimbursed through Medical Assistance and Medicare. Other team members who have been part of the team at some point include vocational support counselors (Lehman et al. 2002), a bookkeeper who provides administration for the team's representative payee program, and an addictions counselor, as well as a variety of trainees including psychiatry residents, social work and psychology interns, and medical, nursing, and occupational therapy students. The team continues to encourage clients to use office-based services and offers multiple groups including a women's group, a men's group, dual-diagnosis groups, an occupational therapy group, and a nursing group. The team has benefited from a HUD-funded Safe Haven, a low-demand shelter for homeless individuals with severe mental illness who are not engaged in treatment (Porterfield 2005), operated through the University of Maryland system, and from the SSI Outreach Project, a SAMHSA-funded program, also operated through the University of Maryland, which can greatly hasten the process of obtaining entitlements for an individual through a process of presumptive disability (Perret 2005). The Baltimore ACT team continues to work to discharge patients, often to traditional community mental health clinics or less intensive case management services within the University of Maryland system. Our experience has been that many individuals can make this transition successfully, and those who do not do well in less intensive services can return to ACT. Of 67 patients who transitioned to less intensive services within the University of Maryland system during a recent 6-year period, 45 had remained in treatment, 8 had returned to ACT services, and the remainder either had left the area or were lost to follow-up (A. Hackman and K. Stowell, "Transitioning ACT Patients to Less Intensive Services." Unpublished manuscript, 2005).

EXAMPLE OF AN ACT TREATMENT PLAN

The ACT team uses individual treatment plans for each patient. These are updated at least quarterly and have goals that are specifically tailored to the needs and wishes of each individual. Figures 5–1 and 5–2 show an initial treatment plan for Mr. D. Although multiple problems were identified, this treatment plan focused on engaging Mr. D with the treatment team. During initial months the team visited Mr. D several times a week at a designated spot in the area where he spent most of his time; at these visits, team members provided Mr. D with drinks, sandwiches, and articles of clothing.

CONCLUSION

The work of the Baltimore ACT team and of other ACT teams serving a homeless population underscores several points. First, there is good evidence that ACT is a treatment model well suited for engaging homeless individuals with severe mental illness. The intensive outreach approach and commitment to addressing whatever needs the client may have works extremely well with a homeless population. Several authors (Dixon et al. 1995; Tsemberis et al. 2000) emphasize the importance of treating the client with respect and providing the services that he or she wants, an approach that included not forcing medications or substance use treatment. This is consistent with the thinking of other writers in that, while ACT is sometimes criticized as coercive (Gomory 2002; Watts and Priebe 2002), it is actually a model of treatment that can be quite consistent with the concepts of empowerment and recovery (Chinman et al. 1999; Mueser et al. 2003). This may be particularly true in a homeless population.

REFERENCES

Aagaar J, Nielsen JA: Experience from the first ACT programme in Denmark, II. Severe mental illness: a register diagnosis. Nord J Psychiatry 58:171–174, 2004

Becker RE, Meisler N, Stormer G, et al: Employment outcomes for clients with severe mental illness in a PACT model replication. Program for Assertive Community Treatment. Psychiatr Serv 50:104–106, 1999

Burns T, Fioritti A, Holloway F, et al: Case management and assertive community treatment in Europe. Psychiatr Serv 52:631–636, 2001

Calsyn RJ, Morse GA, Klinkenberg WD, et al: The impact of assertive community treatment on the social relationships of people who are homeless and mentally ill. Community Ment Health J 34:579–593, 1998

Chinman M, Allende M, Bailey P, et al: Therapeutic agents of assertive community treatment. Psychiatr Q 70:137–162, 1999

Chue P, Tibbo P, Wright E, et al: Client and community services satisfaction with an assertive community treatment subprogram for inner-city clients in Edmonton, Alberta. Can J Psychiatry 49:621–624, 2004

Dixon L: Assertive community treatment: twenty-five years of gold. Psychiatr Serv 51:759–765, 2000

Dixon L, Friedman N, Lehman A: Compliance of homeless mentally ill persons with assertive community treatment. Hosp Community Psychiatry 44:581–583, 1993

Dixon L, Krauss N, Lehman AF: Consumers as service providers: the promise and challenge. Community Ment Health J 30:615–625, 1994

Dixon LB, Krauss N, Kernan E, et al: Modifying the PACT model to serve homeless persons with severe mental illness. Psychiatr Serv 46:684–688, 1995

Dixon L, Hackman A, Lehman A: Consumers as staff in assertive community treatment programs. Adm Policy Ment Health 25:199–208, 1997

Dixon L, Stewart B, Krauss N, et al: The participation of families of homeless persons with severe mental illness in an outreach intervention. Community Ment Health J 34:251–259, 1998

Drake RE, McHugo GJ, Clark RE, et al: Assertive community treatment for patients with co-occurring severe mental illness and substance use disorder: a clinical trial. Am J Orthopsychiatry 68:201–215, 1998

Gomory T: The origins of coercion in Assertive Community Treatment: a review of early publications from the special treatment unit of Mendota State Hospital. Ethical Hum Sci Serv 4:3–16, 2002

Hambridge JA, Rosen A: Assertive community treatment for the seriously mentally ill in suburban Sydney: a programme description and evaluation. Aust N Z J Psychiatry 28:438–445, 1994

Lamberti JS, Weisman R, Faden DI: Forensic assertive community treatment: preventing incarceration of adults with severe mental illness. Psychiatr Serv 55:1285–1293, 2004

Lehman AF, Steinwachs DM: Translating research into practice: the Schizophrenia Patients Outcomes Research Team (PORT) treatment recommendations. Schizophr Bull 24:1–10, 1998

Lehman AF, Dixon LB, Kernan E, et al: A randomized trial of assertive community treatment for homeless persons with severe mental illness. Arch Gen Psychiatry 54:1038–1043, 1997

Lehman AF, Goldberg R, Dixon LB, et al: Improving employment outcomes for persons with severe mental illnesses. Arch Gen Psychiatry 59:165–172, 2002

Lehman AF, Kreyenbuhl J, Buchanan RW, et al: The Schizophrenia Patient Outcomes Research Team (PORT) updated recommendations 2003. Schizophr Bull 30:193–217, 2004

Lim CG, Koh CW, Lee C, et al: Community psychiatry in Singapore: a pilot assertive community treatment (ACT) programme. Ann Acad Med Singapore 34:100–104, 2005

Marx AJ, Test MA, Stein LI: Extrahospital management of severe mental illness: feasibility and effects of social functioning. Arch Gen Psychiatry 29:505–511, 1973

McCoy ML, Roberts DL, Hanrahan P, et al: Jail linkage assertive community treatment services for individuals with mental illnesses. Psychiatr Rehabil J 27:243–250, 2004

McFarlane WR: FACT: integrating family psychoeducation and assertive community treatment. Adm Policy Ment Health 25:191–198, 1997

McFarlane WR, Stastny P, Deakins S: Family-aided assertive community treatment: a comprehensive rehabilitation and intensive case management approach for persons with schizophrenic disorders. New Dir Ment Health Serv 53:43–54, 1992

McFarlane WR, Dushay RA, Stastny P, et al: A comparison of two levels of family-aided assertive community treatment. Psychiatr Serv 47:744–750, 1996

McGrew JH, Bond GR: The association between program characteristics and service delivery in assertive community treatment. Adm Policy Ment Health 25:175–189, 1997

McGuire JF, Rosenheck RA: Criminal history as a prognostic indicator in the treatment of homeless people with severe mental illness. Psychiatr Serv 55:42–48, 2004

McHugo GJ, Drake RE, Teague GB, et al: Fidelity to assertive community treatment and client outcomes in the New Hampshire dual disorders study. Psychiatr Serv 50:818–824, 1999

Meisler N, Blankertz L, Santos AB, et al: Impact of assertive community treatment on homeless persons with co-occurring severe psychiatric and substance use disorders. Community Ment Health J 33:113–122, 1997

Morse GA, Calsyn RJ, Allen G, et al: Experimental comparison of the effects of three treatment programs for homeless mentally ill people. Hosp Community Psychiatry 43:1005–1010, 1992

Morse GA, Calsyn RJ, Klinkenberg WD, et al: An experimental comparison of three types of case management for homeless mentally ill persons. Psychiatr Serv 48:497–503, 1997

Mueser KT, Torrey WC, Lynde D, et al: Implementing evidence-based practices for people with severe mental illness. Behav Modif 27:387–411, 2003

Perret Y: The Maryland SSI Outreach Project Baltimore Maryland. National Alliance to End Homelessness Web site. Available at: http://www.endhomelessness.org/best/mdssioutrch.htm. Accessed May 19, 2005.

Porterfield D: Planning, designing, siting and financing safe haven housing, in In From the Cold: Safe Havens for Homeless People. Tool Kit, U.S. Department of Housing and Urban Development Homes and Communities Web site. Available at: http://www.hud.gov/offices/cpd/homeless/library/havens/ch2.pdf. Accessed May 19, 2005.

Priebe S, Fakhoury W, Watts J, et al: Assertive outreach teams in London: patient characteristics and outcomes. Pan-London Assertive Outreach Study, part 3. Br J Psychiatry 183:148–154, 2003

Randolph F, Blasinsky M, Morrissey JP, et al: Overview of the ACCESS program. ACCESS National Evaluation Team. Psychiatr Serv 53:945–948, 2002

Rosenheck RA, Dennis D: Time-limited assertive community treatment for homeless persons with severe mental illness. Arch Gen Psychiatry 58:1073–1080, 2001

Rosenheck RA, Neale MS: Therapeutic limit setting and six-month outcomes in a Veterans Affairs assertive community treatment program. Psychiatr Serv 55:139–144, 2004

Stein LI, Santos AB: Assertive Community Treatment of Persons With Severe Mental Illness. New York, WW Norton, 1998

Teague GB, Drake RE, Ackerson TH: Evaluating use of continuous treatment teams for persons with mental illness and substance abuse. Psychiatr Serv 46:689–695, 1995

Test MA, Stein LI: Alternative to mental hospital treatment, III: social cost. Arch Gen Psychiatry 37:409–412, 1980

Tsemberis S, Eisenberg RF: Pathways to housing: supported housing for street-dwelling homeless individuals with psychiatric disabilities. Psychiatr Serv 51:487–493, 2000

Tyrer P, Simmonds S: Treatment models for those with severe mental illness and co-morbid personality disorder. Br J Psychiatry Suppl 44:S15–S18, 2003

Watts J, Priebe S: A phenomenological account of users' experiences of assertive community treatment. Bioethics 16:439–454, 2002

Weisbrod MA, Test MA, Stein LI: Alternative to mental hospital treatment, II: economic benefit and cost analysis. Arch Gen Psychiatry 37:400–405, 1980

Zaluska M, Suchecka D, Traczewska Z, et al: Implementation of social services for the chronically mentally ill in a Polish mental health district: consequences for service use and costs. J Ment Health Policy Econ 8:37–44, 2005

Chapter 6

HOUSING

Ralph Aquila, M.D.
John Kelleher
Thomas Sweet

Once a homeless person is engaged into treatment, it is essential to bring resources to that person in order to retain him or her in a rehabilitation process and to foster a sense of recovery. In this chapter, while telling one person's story, we will describe how a move into housing, with the use of the "rehabilitation alliance" approach, serves recovery and rehabilitation. First, Jack's presentation:

> Jack was a 63-year-old single Caucasian who presented to us homeless, psychotic, and with alcohol abuse. He had an erratic treatment history with repeated episodes of treatment nonadherence. Although he had technically been a member of our clubhouse program for 30 years, he had been out of any treatment for over 12 months. Jack was viewed as an ever more difficult management problem. His bipolar disorder and drinking increased his irritability and hostility, and he often threatened people with harm. Because of money mismanagement, he was also now living on the street, despite having been housed in the past through various of our clubhouse's programs.

A person with serious and persistent mental illness traditionally has been viewed as too disabled to participate in mainstream society, and this is magnified with homelessness. To live independently, hold down a job, have a circle of friends, and live a happy and productive life was considered beyond such a person's functional capacities (Harding and Zahniser 1994). Rather, it was believed that the person needed prolonged care. Although we believe this notion is changing, homelessness complicates the recovery process. For example, the realities of living on the street severely compromise a person's ability to store belongings and to do even basic scheduling, affecting medication adherence among other things. It is well known that over the last 25 years, there has been a culture change among those with serious mental illness; a patient discharged from long-term hospitalization is very different from a young person with schizophrenia who has had multiple inpatient acute stays while never seeing a state hospital (Pepper et al. 1981). Not having been in a hospital center leads to greater mistrust of medical-psychiatric personnel. With the younger patients or those who have been homeless for many years, this can lead to greater difficulty in the initial engagement process. Once again, this alienation is complicated by homelessness, making integration more difficult. Mental illness in and of itself is stigmatizing, but when you are homeless the stigma is compounded. For many homeless persons, not having access to showers and other means of personal hygiene creates that "homeless look." There is a greater tendency for the public to avoid people who have that appearance. Therefore, symptoms such as paranoia become even more accentuated.

> Both his psychiatrist and his social worker, a senior program administrator, made numerous attempts to engage Jack. Early on there was little progress, but finally he agreed to enter supervised housing, start medication, and return to Fountain House more consistently. His condition stabilized with an atypical antipsychotic agent, which he said was the first tolerable medication he had ever taken. We reintroduced him to the clubhouse and offered him competitive employment as a receptionist and clerical worker. He jumped at the opportunity. His personal charm, motivation, and sense of organization enabled him to move ahead. The combination of psychiatric care with rehabilitation was a turning point in this man's life.

In achieving this level of recovery, it is necessary to take a step back and assess the person for who he or she is, identifying potential strengths. These include the capacity to become better organized through managing one's own money and paying bills on time, maintaining personal hygiene, and shopping and cooking. The degree to which a person's recovery leads to improved functional abilities informs the kind of housing supports he or she will need at the time of gaining access to a place to live.

HOUSING MODELS

Because affordable housing is scarce in many areas, housing opportunities often are subject to resource allocation, with access to a bed dependent on the advocacy of the referring provider. Nonetheless, some localities have developed housing management criteria for determining the placement of a mentally ill homeless people. For example, the New York City Human Resources Administration has defined and allocated two distinct levels of housing based on reported intensity of service needs (New York/New York III 2005), regardless of whether the housing is congregate or scatter-site in format.

These housing levels are functionally divided into two basic categories: "supervised" to "supportive," that is, from highly to minimally structured in terms of staff and on-site services. Within these two housing categories, there is further variation in service intensity and structure, and this is often derived from the culture of individual housing programs themselves. This requires the psychiatric clinician to be flexible in his or her role.

For example, for homeless patients in the early recovery stages, close assistance with personal hygiene management and with medication supervision may be essential, as may intensive interventions (based on either harm reduction or abstinence) toward eventual sobriety. This prevents illness exacerbation, which has traditionally been viewed as being in the nature of psychiatric illness, even though, in the great majority of cases, it is actually based on stopping medication or on alcohol and substance use.

> In Jack's situation, the rehabilitation team opted for a transitional stay in a highly supervised level of housing, allowing him to consolidate functional gains with additional environmental supports. He followed this with permanent supportive-level housing based on his medication adherence and his ability to budget his funds and attend sobriety meetings. The psychiatrist was particularly active during Jack's transitional housing tenure. After careful construction of a treatment relationship, the use of an atypical antipsychotic agent helped Jack with spontaneous adherence in that its side effects, unlike those of first-generation antipsychotics, did not appear to exacerbate Jack's depression or challenge his alertness and motor coordination. Importantly, also integral to later sustaining treatment was the notion that he could have gainful employment.

As recovery progresses and illness self-management skills increase, the level of supervision tapers accordingly (Anthony and Farkas 1982) and the psychiatric clinician increasingly focuses his or her work on supporting recovery initiatives led by the rest of the rehabilitation treatment team, both within and beyond the walls of the community residence.

It is noteworthy, however, that few data exist regarding the types of supports best suited for persons at different stages of recovery (McQuistion et al. 2003). In fact, some may assert that a person should be housed as soon as possible, regardless of illness severity and availability of a concomitant level of supervisory support. In our view, that is philosophically appealing, but in practice it may present problems for maintaining housing stability. Alternatively, some programs employ an approach of rapid housing even for the most impaired homeless people, but also provide mobile community treatment supports in a flexible way to optimize housing tenure. Tsemberis and Eisenberg (2000) examined one such model that provided robust housing tenure compared with more traditional housing formats.

Regardless of format, staff is important in supervised/supportive housing. The training of staff generally varies from paraprofessional to master's-degree level. Medical professionals are rarely present, and nursing staff can be of great benefit in medication management, enabling the psychiatric clinician to have more flexibility in titrating medications and switching regimens. Nursing can also help identify and assess medical comorbidities. With better-integrated services in housing programs and resultant greater success in achieving psychiatric stability and treatment engagement, patients are also more accessible to primary care, yielding a greater opportunity to diagnose and treat chronic medical conditions such as diabetes mellitus, hypertension, and chronic obstructive pulmonary disease (Breakey et al. 1989).

In working in housing, psychiatrists have acquired skills in both traditional and less traditional interventions. Traditional interventions consist of diagnostics, psychosocial assessment, and psychopharmacology. Less traditional skills often involve working with staff: teaching inexperienced collaborating staff and developing techniques attuned to seeing patients in a natural setting—their home, rather than a hospital or clinic. This vital opportunity not only helps the clinician develop an egalitarian approach to patient care but also enables access to subtle clinical information, for example, detecting early signs of illness exacerbation or chemical-dependency relapse. To this end especially, everyone in the building can be helpful, including maintenance staff who may alert the psychiatrist to psychotic behavior, as well as other residents who are concerned about their neighbors and friends.

ESTABLISHING PERMANENT HOUSING: A SUCCESSFUL MODEL

Regardless of the intensity of supervision, it is important to remain focused on the goals of living: a nice place to live (independence), something meaningful to do (competitive employment), and a meaningful social network (friends and family). An approach in reaching these goals is to conceptualize a multidisciplinary team with the consumer at its center. The rest of the team consists of a psychiatrist, a social worker, possibly a nurse, and sometimes a landlord or employer (Aquila et al. 1999). When the team and the individual meet together, the interaction is based on assessing with the person where he or she is on the continuum of recovery. For example, questions are asked about how the person is doing as a clubhouse member or at his or her job placement. By addressing these issues, we are also able either directly or indirectly to elicit the member's symptoms. Therapeutically, it makes an important difference to address recent positive accomplishments, as opposed to merely focusing on pathology or problems with behavior.

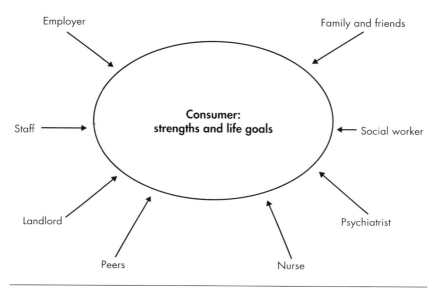

FIGURE 6–1. Supportive housing clubhouse model: the rehabilitation alliance.

This approach, also called the *rehabilitation alliance,* is employed at Fountain House, a community-based rehabilitation organization that originated the "clubhouse" model in 1948 (Fountain House 2005). Figure 6–1 illustrates the structure of this model. Currently, 350 such clubhouses exist worldwide, and the essence of membership in these programs is expressed in four "guaranteed rights" that build on members' wellness: 1) a place to come to and belong; 2) meaningful work; 3) meaningful relationships; and 4) a place to return to through lifetime membership (Beard et al. 1982). If stable housing is added to these rights, the ingredients of recovery may be considered nearly complete (see Figure 6–2).

In the late 1990s, Fountain House was very successful in reaching out to homeless people with serious mental illness. The work consisted of a clubhouse outreach team engaging and encouraging people to come to its clinic (purposely based in a storefront setting) to get a meal, a shower, and medical and psychiatric services. Potential clubhouse members who were homeless were then invited on a tour of Fountain House, with a subsequent invitation to become a Fountain House member. Through storefront services, or at Fountain House itself, members are engaged toward housing, either transitional or permanent.

The Rehabilitation Alliance

The doctor-patient relationship has historically been seen as a key to success in the treatment of illness and an important factor in successful rehabilitation.

Pathway to recovery

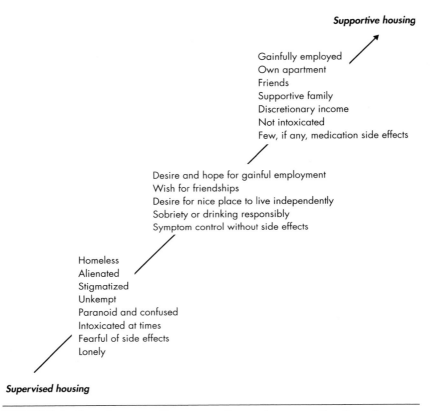

Supportive housing

Gainfully employed
Own apartment
Friends
Supportive family
Discretionary income
Not intoxicated
Few, if any, medication side effects

Desire and hope for gainful employment
Wish for friendships
Desire for nice place to live independently
Sobriety or drinking responsibly
Symptom control without side effects

Homeless
Alienated
Stigmatized
Unkempt
Paranoid and confused
Intoxicated at times
Fearful of side effects
Lonely

Supervised housing

FIGURE 6–2.   Process of recovery through supportive housing.

The traditional "therapeutic alliance," however, has often been insufficient in meeting the needs of persons with serious and persistent mental illness (Gutheil and Havens 1979), with nonadherence being a major culprit. Although the disorder's severity or lack of response to an adequate therapeutic regimen also poses a serious challenge, the therapeutic alliance is often adversely affected by experience within the mental health system. Brief, impersonal encounters, limited shared diagnostic information, a focus on psychopathology and symptom management, narrow-vision recovery possibilities, lack of community support and opportunity, isolation among service providers—all these factors can combine to avoid focusing on life goals, strengths, hopes, persistence, creativity, courage, and the compassion that are essential ingredients for building and maintaining alliances.

As noted, the rehabilitation alliance in its most concrete form refers to a team consisting of the consumer, the psychiatrist, and staff or another peer. However, this alliance actually consists of the network of relationships that develop over time to support people with disabilities in their pursuit of recovery. It therefore also includes family and friends and, in a more general way, employers and landlords. The basis of this alliance is the mutual respect, trust, and seriousness of purpose that develop among these people as they engage each other, stabilizing, restoring, and enhancing the ability of the disabled person to function consistently, regain control of his or her life, and become a valued and contributing member of the community (Gutheil and Havens 1979). The rehabilitation alliance focuses on strengths and life goals; it acknowledges problems and clinical needs. It supports hope, yet it does not deny pain and sorrow. It is persistent; it recognizes the nonlinear nature of the recovery process. It is creative in that it identifies opportunities for people to find their diverse pathways. It is courageous; it encourages risk-taking one step at a time. It is compassionate, practical, and humane. As the work unfolds, the alliance is challenged and strengthened. In a remarkable way, it invites all participants to grow, to co-evolve. Although the primary focus is on the member, this growth process also affects the other participants in important ways.

Implications for Practice

The rehabilitation alliance differs from other models with respect to the role that each participant assumes. The member evolves from being a passive recipient of services to a co-team leader: an active participant in the treatment process. The individual's life goals become primary to the rehabilitation process; the treatment of symptoms as an end unto itself disappears. Although the purpose of the rehabilitation alliance is to support the recovery, clearly the interaction also benefits the other participants. Clinicians grow professionally and personally when they perceive the intelligence and personality that emerge from their patients as the illness is controlled and as they cultivate the multifaceted rehabilitation alliance. The clinician's role also broadens from that of service provider to collaborator in the joint treatment-rehabilitation plan. This broadening is only possible when the myth that people with serious and persistent mental illness cannot work is dispelled (McCrory 1991).

The model is most effective when it is part of a formal rehabilitation program, but it can also be effective in standalone housing programs. Fundamentally, among staff, the process begins with the psychiatrist and other key professionals who believe that a person, no matter how ill, can recover and improve his or her lot in life, so that their focus becomes making the *person* better, not just relieving symptoms. This message then must be transmitted to the rest of the housing staff. From the patient's vantage point, the same process begins with the formulation of specific personal goals, usually concerning greater independence followed by employment or a return to education.

One final point needs to be made. The nature of participation in the clubhouse community is based on the individual's functioning as a generalist rather than a specialist. When a person enters the clubhouse as a trained psychiatrist or lawyer, for example, the individual and the community as a whole need to perceive him or her not in terms of that specialty, but rather as a generalist, a team member. Likewise, both the community and each individual need to know the person by name (Joan, Sam, or Leslie), not as "a lawyer" or "a psychiatrist." Although such a value is easy to identify, making it a working perception is another, more difficult matter. We believe that much progress has been made; however, much more needs to be done in habilitating and humanizing the specialist.

REFERENCES

Anthony WA, Farkas M: A client outcome planning model for assessing psychiatric rehabilitation interventions. Schizophr Bull 8:13–38, 1982

Aquila R, Santos G, Malamud T, et al: The rehabilitation alliance in practice: the clubhouse connection. Psychiatr Rehabil J 23:19–23, 1999

Beard JH, Propst RN, Malamud TJ: The Fountain House model of psychosocial rehabilitation. Psychosocial Rehabilitation Journal 5:47–53, 1982

Breakey WR, Fischer PJ, Kramer M, et al: Health and mental health problems of homeless men and women in Baltimore. JAMA 262:1352–1357, 1989

Fountain House: Who We Are. Available at: http://www.fountainhouse.org/moxie/who. Accessed December 30, 2005.

Gutheil TG, Havens LL: The therapeutic alliance: contemporary meanings and confusion. Int Rev Psychoanal 467–481, 1979

Harding CM, Zahniser JH: Empirical correction of seven myths about schizophrenia with implications for treatment. Acta Psychiatr Scand Suppl 90:140–146, 1994

McCrory DJ: The rehabilitation alliance. Journal of Vocational Rehabilitation 1:58–66, 1991

McQuistion HL, Finnerty M, Hirschowitz J, et al: Challenges for psychiatry in serving homeless people with psychiatric disorders. Psychiatr Serv 54: 669–676, 2003

New York/New York III Agreement: Joint housing initiative. The City of New York and the State of New York, 2005

Pepper B, Kirshner MC, Ryglewicz H: The young adult chronic patient: overview of a population. Hosp Community Psychiatry 32:463–469, 1981 [reprinted in: Psychiatr Serv 51:996–1000, 2000]

Tsemberis S, Eisenberg RF: Pathways to Housing: supported housing for street-dwelling homeless individuals with psychiatric disabilities. Psychiatr Serv 51:487–493, 2000

Chapter 7

MOBILE CRISIS TEAMS

Anthony T. Ng, M.D.

A shelter manager with minimal mental health training telephoned a referral to the Mobile Crisis Team (MCT) to see a homeless woman in her 50s. The shelter manager reported that the woman had been acting "bizarre and paranoid" and was "talking to herself." He was afraid to confront her because of his fear that she would become violent. He said she had a psychiatric history and her case was being followed at a neighborhood mental health clinic, but he did not know who her case manager was. He was not sure if the woman had any weapons.

INTRODUCTION: THE ROLE OF MOBILE CRISIS TEAMS

Before addressing this case in detail, it is useful to put mobile crisis services into context. Mobile crisis teams are integral to emergency psychiatric services (Gillig 1993; Zealberg et al. 1993). Outreach is an important component of MCT work and in reference to both process and outcome. MCT, as part of crisis stabilization, focuses on creating and building rapport and trust and eventually engaging clients in necessary services, a process that takes from weeks to months, sometimes years, to accomplish (Interagency Council on the Homeless 1991; McMurray-Avila 1997; Ng and McQuistion 2004). Some studies have shown MCT to be cost-effective and to decrease hospitalization rates (Bengelsdorf et al. 1993; Guo et al. 2001; Scott et al. 2000; Zealberg 1993), although little empirical research is available about its efficacy in preventing rehospitalization (Geller et al. 1995). There is also a scarcity of literature available to the MCT clinician on conducting the practical aspects of mobile crisis outreach, such as guides to locating and engaging clients.

For the MCT to be an effective intervention in any forum, there must be an appreciation of both the extrinsic and intrinsic influences on any MCT and of the complex relationships between them (Ng 2004). Extrinsic challenges include working conditions and interaction with the mental health system. Because of their close relationship to actual clinical work, intrinsic influences are most relevant to this chapter. These influences primarily refer to intrateam issues, including clinician training and attitudes, individual personalities, and how team members interact and achieve the most efficient team structure and job satisfaction.

MCT Composition and Support

In my view, successful outreach clinicians have personal characteristics such as empathy, a collaborative approach, respect for personal autonomy, and the ability to listen on varying social and psychological levels to the client (Scott 2000). However, MCT clinicians also have an ability to work in settings that are fluid, particularly when interacting with the homeless population, requiring flexibility and creativity. MCT clinicians need to be able to work in a team and relate with professionals of varying disciplines as well as lay individuals. One particularly important interaction is with law enforcement, which frequently partners with MCTs in the context of involuntary interventions. Well-developed mobile crisis teams are actively engaged with local law enforcement, collegially through cross-training efforts and administratively through formal collaborative memoranda of understanding or with the support of their government funding agencies.

MCT clinicians must also appreciate and tolerate the potential lack of control and the clinical limitations and challenges that are present in any MCT intervention. An effective MCT is not only based on individual clinician skills, but also includes clinical experience and life experiences. Like all clinicians, those who work in MCT will have personal experiences and predisposing views and attitudes—cultural, religious, or uniquely personal—that shape the therapeutic work in which outreach clinicians engage (Comas-Diaz 1991; Goering et al. 1992; Minrath 1985; Shechter 1992). Both individual MCT clinicians and MCT program directors must develop an awareness of how those views and attitudes can influence their work and cultivate diversity to enhance the effectiveness of the team. Mobile crisis teamwork is intimate: clinicians travel together and eat together, and they may share their personal lives with each other (Ng and McQuistion 2004). Effective team dynamics can decrease clinical and professional isolation, enhance safety, provide diverse expertise both clinically and culturally, prevent splitting between client and staff, and enhance MCT clinical intervention overall. The team personality guides how clinical interventions are conducted. Ongoing review of mission, advocacy and promotion of staff wellness, and periodic evaluations of overall performance support the team personality and its individual members. These procedures minimize burnout, the signs of which include staff turnover, decreased productivity, and organizational discord—all of which affect program performance.

Another mechanism to enhance the morale and mission of MCT is its use as a training site, creating mentorship roles for staff. MCT offers an opportunity for students and trainees to acquire unique assessment and engagement skills in working with mentally ill homeless people, presenting trainees with real frontline clinical work in which they manage both practical and clinical needs. Students and trainees also learn teamwork and how to integrate their knowledge into nontraditional clinical formats.

MAKING A DIAGNOSIS IN THE SETTING: ROLE OF THE MOBILE CRISIS TEAM

An important component of any successful MCT intervention begins at the referral process. Referrals regarding homeless persons often come from several sources, including the current medical or psychiatric treatment team, family, service agencies, the police, and the court system. It is important that the MCT obtain as much information as possible to formulate an effective plan. Specifically, why is the person being referred? What is the reason for the referral: neglect in self-care, threat to others, or treatment noncompliance? It is important to discern secondary reasons for referral, too. MCT referrals may be made for social as well as psychiatric reasons. For example, a stated reason for referral of a homeless individual at a shelter may be to evaluate agitation, but a secondary reason may be to remove the individual from the shelter for disruptive behavior. It is important to clarify from the referral source the intervention that is requested, for instance, crisis stabilization or placement into a higher level of care such as hospitalization.

Detailed demographic and descriptive information about the person to be evaluated should be obtained. This should include age, gender, location, and time of day to best reach both the individual and the referral source, as well as the homeless person's physical appearance—what the person is wearing or what sort of belongings he or she may have.

Clearly, relevant past psychiatric, substance use, and medical history must be ascertained in the referral process. The MCT referral also should include the presence of any potential physical disabilities (such as limited mobility) or sensory disabilities that may affect the MCT intervention. For example, does the individual use ambulatory aids or service animals? Is the person's hearing impaired, necessitating sign language interpreting?

UNIQUE ASPECTS OF THE MOBILE CRISIS TEAM SETTING

Before an MCT is actually dispatched, it is important to identify and plan potential interventions. Whereas some referrals may require more educational and resource-oriented interventions, some require acute intervention such as police and emergency medical services. When taking an MCT referral, the intake clinician should inquire about safety-related issues such as whether the person is agitated or has the potential for harm to self and others. Although physical acting-out is not common, dangerous situations are still relatively frequent (Pochard et al. 1998). Other safety concerns include access to weapons, physical barricades that can prevent entry or interaction, presence of animals such as dogs, presence of infectious illness such as active tuberculosis, and self-care issues such as lice and scabies.

Instructions should be given to the referral source about what to do until the MCT arrives, including strategies to temporarily stabilize the situation. It is important that the referral source and the MCT exchange contact numbers in case the referral information changes.

Before any MCT assessment, the team must discuss strategies to conduct the assessment, even if the referral seems uncomplicated. Using the information obtained in the referral process, MCT members should identify the goals of its interventions, addressing both the primary and secondary reasons for referral. Alternative goals should be identified in the event that the clinical presentation is different from that obtained during the referral process. For example, the referred individual may be more impaired and in greater distress than originally presented. In such instances, MCT members should determine the threshold for involuntary transport to an emergency room. As in the identification of intervention goals for any MCT referral, it is important that there be consensus regarding this threshold within the MCT.

Through the referral process, MCT members determine the approach to the client and his or her environment. Because MCT interventions with homeless people are often conducted on the street, in shelters, and in other atypical settings, team members must appreciate special issues presented by these environments. This includes the presence of any additional people at the location who might aid or hinder the crisis intervention. For example, the MCT may want to provide as much privacy as possible for a street homeless person, to avoid unnecessary attention and well-meaning but inappropriate involvement by passersby. One instance is recalled in which MCT members were accosted by people on the street for "bothering" a homeless elderly man. This type of situation extends to a need for the MCT to decide whether the actual location for contact with the referred person is conducive to MCT intervention, thus deciding what precautions are necessary to see the client. Observation of the environment can help to mitigate any potential risk factors external to the client-clinician interaction. In another instance, an MCT member was a victim of an attempted robbery at a bus station while the team was evaluating a client. Under these circumstances, one approach is to identify a lead clinician interacting primarily with the client, with a second clinician monitoring the environment but assisting the lead clinician as necessary.

> After receiving the referral, the MCT clinicians discussed the desired outcome of the intervention with the shelter manager. The manager expressed frustration at the woman's behavior and a desire to have her "taken away to a hospital." He stated the woman worried him and other residents.
> Before the MCT was dispatched, safety issues were clarified, including the best time to visit and whether there was any risk of the presence of animals or weapons. The team discussed how to approach the homeless woman if she showed fear of the team. The MCT discussed with the referral source the availability of various treatment outcomes that could be explored in addition to hospitalization. They also planned for the possibility of emergency hospitalization, deciding how the referral would be initiated and by which clinician. On the basis of the information obtained, the MCT dispatched two clinicians: a female psychiatrist and a male social worker. The psychiatrist evaluated the woman's level of dangerousness and determined whether emergency hospitalization was needed. The social worker was available to implement nonhospitalization referrals if appropriate.

MCTs often receive multiple referrals, and because resources and personnel are limited, they need to prioritize and triage referrals. Triage should take into account several factors. The most important are *urgency* and *acuity*. Urgency and acuity are based on risk of threat to self and others, level of distress, and impairment. However, other factors may influence urgency and acuity. For example: Are there any available supports for the homeless person until MCT intervention is possible? Are the means of harm readily available, such as firearms, knives, or pills for overdose? Whether or not the client is at the location will be important also because it may indicate the level of mobility of the client, as well as the level of urgency and acuity. For example, if an agitated client at a quiet street corner is moving toward a heavy traffic area, then psychiatric intervention by the outreach team may be more urgent and may even warrant intervention of law enforcement.

For visits to domiciled persons, the referred person normally is notified by telephone that an MCT intervention will occur. This may not be possible in the case of a homeless person, but if the individual is in a shelter he or she should be oriented, if at all possible, to who made the referral, how the MCT visit will be conducted, how many MCT clinicians will arrive, and what their credentials are. Shelter operators should also be encouraged to elicit the indi-

vidual's concerns about the MCT visits. This can allow the individual to prepare for the visit and invoke coping strategies such as sitting in a quiet area
or conversing with a trusted staff member.

In MCT assessment, observational findings can be particularly important, particularly when the person is not productive in his or her verbal behavior. Does body language communicate ease, or does it convey tension and
volatility, with threatening or defensive posturing, hands clenched, and rest-
lessness? Although such signs may be attributable to reasons such as medication side effects (which themselves can exacerbate distress), clinicians should
be mindful of all behavioral clues to a person's condition. Moreover, MCT
clinicians should take the opportunity to use the person's physical environment to assess evidence of current level of self-care. Distress may be evi-
denced by how disheveled the individual or the environment is, or even by
how unusually tidy things look. During one encounter, an MCT noted that
a person with paranoid ideation had an extremely tidy area around her in a
shelter—only to learn later that she scrubbed the area constantly with bleach
to keep away nonexistent snakes. Body language also is important.

> On MCT assessment, the woman was acting bizarrely in the hallway of the
> shelter. The team noted that she was guarded in her attitude and affect, asking
> who they were and why they were after her. After spending some time ex-
> plaining who they were, the MCT staff were able to persuade the woman to
> talk to them in her room. One of the team's clinicians talked to the woman
> while the other stayed a bit behind to observe the shelter environment. The
> woman was noted to be internally preoccupied. During course of assessment,
> the MCT discovered that she had missed several appointments at a commu-
> nity mental health center because she said someone had yelled at her and she
> believed that person might be trying to harm her. She stopped going, and
> when she tried to contact her case manager and got no response, she surmised
> that her case manager had conspired with the person who yelled at her. Her
> antipsychotic medication prescription had not been renewed, and as a result
> her condition was exacerbated.

A primary aim of MCT is stabilization. Unlike traditional office settings,
MCT interventions occur in atypical environments—sometimes with a need
for rapid resolution, depending on the nature of the crisis. It is important during
the assessment to acquire as much information as possible, obtaining enough
data to afford clinical definitions addressing MCT intervention goals. As noted
concerning environmental assessment, it is important to appreciate that crisis
stabilization involves more than the client alone. MCT clinicians need to assess
systemic issues that may have precipitated or mitigated the crisis. For example,
a homeless person may be agitated because he or she is in an overcrowded shelter and had been accosted by other shelter residents. Consultation with shelter
staff regarding the person's safety is indicated under such circumstances.

DEVELOPMENT OF A TREATMENT PLAN BY THE MOBILE CRISIS TEAM

> After assessing the homeless woman, the MCT clinicians determined that although her psychiatric disorder had exacerbated, she was not dangerous to herself or other people; therefore, referral for involuntary hospitalization was deferred. The team members expressed to the woman their concerns for her wellbeing and asked if there was anything they could do. They learned that she had an overall positive relationship with the mental health center, so they stressed the importance of her reconnecting with that clinic. Because the MCT clinicians were able to develop rapport with her, they asked the woman if she would feel safer if they escorted her to the clinic to make sure she would be safe. The woman voluntarily agreed to the escort in order to meet with a member of her treatment team. Explaining to the woman that the shelter manager was concerned about her, the MCT received her permission to speak with the shelter manager about the plan to reconnect her to the mental health center. The MCT also provided psychoeducation to the shelter manager and supported his concern about the woman's illness.

Devising an intervention plan requires eliciting the patient's input, and the patient's goals must drive its design. The planning may involve honest discussions about the need to negotiate short-term objectives en route to addressing presently unrealistic goals. Additionally, during these discussions, resources should be identified and service liaisons made so that interventions by the MCT can be effective. Both traditional and nontraditional supports for the person should be integrated into the plan insofar as the mentally ill homeless person perceives them as helpful. Once an intervention plan is devised, it is also important to establish a timeline to encourage adherence with the treatment plan. The MCT should remain available for follow-up visits to optimize success, sometimes offering medication monitoring pending connection with more traditional services. It is also crucial that the relevant referral source, such as the client's treatment team, be informed of the treatment plan, timelines, and alternative strategies should the plan break down.

It should be the goal of any MCT intervention to avoid hospitalization. Alternative and less restrictive interventions should be explored, including intensified case management, repeated MCT visits, or day hospital or crisis-residence referrals. However, psychiatric hospitalization is at times warranted. If hospitalization is being considered at the time of referral, a plan should be made in advance. Once the MCT is on the scene and has confirmed an imminent danger, it is an error to inform the agitated individual, before police and emergency medical services arrive, that he or she will be involuntarily transported to a hospital. This can result in increased agitation and risk of violence. If MCT clinicians determine that an extended interaction with the person may result in increased risks of violence or flight, there are several options for how to proceed. One approach is for MCT clinicians to conclude the visit without informing the individual of the plan, then contact police and emergency medical services away from the site. A lead MCT clinician may remain with or near the homeless person while another clinician makes the calls for backup. If a mentally ill homeless person leaves the location before police arrive, an MCT clinician may follow the person if this can be done in a way that is safe for both the individual and the clinician, remaining in contact with the team so that police can be directed to the person's new location.

> The MCT also learned from the woman that she was not happy at the shelter. Other residents had victimized her. She was also having problems obtaining entitlements; the mental health center was her representative payee, and because she had not been keeping appointments, she had not received any financial assistance. With her permission, the MCT contacted her treatment team at the psychiatric clinic. The team learned that the woman's regular case manager had been transferred abruptly and that follow-up had not occurred after the patient failed to show for her scheduled appointment with the new case manager. The MCT contacted the new case manager and escorted the patient to the clinic the next day. Additionally, the MCT discussed with her case manager the team's findings and its recommendations regarding other needs. These included housing, more intensive outpatient monitoring, and the need for MCT on-site and telephone follow-ups to continue until the patient had been reliably reconnected with the mental health center.

ACCESS TO ENTITLEMENTS: ROLE OF THE MOBILE CRISIS TEAM

Some of the factors that place mentally ill homeless persons at risk for repeated illness exacerbation are psychiatrically based, such as treatment nonadherence. However, many of the risk factors for worsening of mental illness are socially related—the most dramatic of these being unavailable, unsafe, or poorly maintained housing. Other such factors include loss of benefits, ongoing discord in relationships, and poor access to medical care. MCT clinicians must know how to broker access to these resources and how to use a "wraparound" approach that may involve collateral social support, social services, and other health services in crisis stabilization, to include both traditional and nontraditional supports (i.e., faith-based supports, social services, other homeless clients). The MCT often becomes the link that ensures a degree of service continuity and comprehensiveness for the mentally ill homeless person.

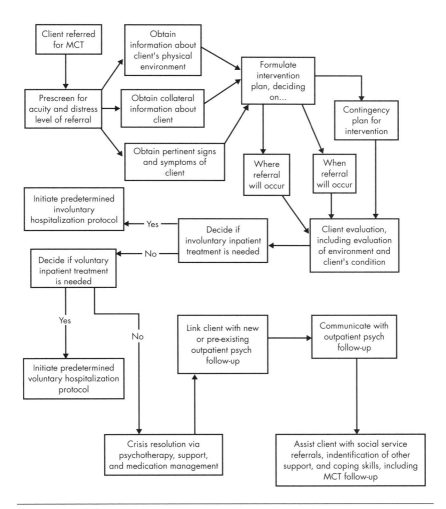

FIGURE 7–1. Flowchart of treatment: a mobile crisis team (MCT) approach to homeless mentally ill persons.

CONCLUSION

MCTs provide unique opportunities for clinicians to work successfully with a challenging segment of the community, the mentally ill homeless population. Although MCT work with homeless people is challenging, it can also be extremely rewarding. Clinicians have the potential to help mentally ill homeless persons who have not responded well to more traditional treatment. The practical paradigm offered in this chapter (see Figure 7–1) will serve clinician skill-building, stimulate discussion on the dynamic of effective mobile crisis work, and encourage closer examination of the effectiveness of a mobile crisis approach in working with mentally ill homeless persons.

REFERENCES

Bengelsdorf H, Church JO, Kaye RA, et al: The cost effectiveness of crisis intervention: admission diversion savings can offset the high cost of service. J Nerv Ment Dis 181:757–762, 1993

Comas-Diaz L, Jacobsen FM: Ethnocultural transference and countertransference in the therapeutic dyad. Am J Orthopsychiatry 61:392–402, 1991

Geller JL, Fisher WH, McDermeit M: A national survey of mobile crisis services and their evaluation. Psychiatr Serv 46:893–897, 1995

Gillig P: The spectrum of mobile outreach and its role in the emergency service. New Dir Ment Health Serv 67:13–21, 1993

Goering P, Wasylenki D, Onge MS, et al: Gender differences among clients of a case management program for the homeless. Hosp Community Psychiatry 43:160–165, 1992

Guo S, Biegel DE, Johnsen JA, et al: Assessing the impact of community-based mobile crisis services on preventing hospitalization. Psychiatr Serv 52:223–228, 2001

Interagency Council on the Homeless: Reaching Out: A Guide for Service Providers. Washington, DC, Interagency Council on the Homeless, 1991

McMurray-Avila M: Organizing Health Services for Homeless People: A Practical Guide. Nashville, TN, National Health Care for the Homeless Council, 1997

Minrath M: Breaking the race barrier. J Psychosoc Nurs Ment Health Serv 23:19–24, 1985

Ng AT, McQuistion HL: Outreach to the homeless: craft, science and future implication. J Psychiatr Pract 10:95–105, 2004

Pochard F, Robin M, Regel I, et al: [Security and home emergency psychiatric interventions] (French). Encephale 24:324–329, 1998

Scott RL: Evaluation of a mobile crisis program: effectiveness, efficiency, and consumer satisfaction. Psychiatr Serv 51:1153–1156, 2000

Shechter RA: Voice of hidden minority: identification and countertransference in the cross-cultural working alliance. Am J Psychoanal 52:339–349, 1992

Zealberg JJ, Santos AB, Fisher RK: Benefits of mobile crisis programs. Hosp Community Psychiatry 44:16–17, 1993

Chapter 8

PSYCHIATRIC EMERGENCY SERVICES

Avrim Fishkind, M.D.
Scott Zeller, M.D.

$\mathbf{P}$olice are summoned to a busy intersection on a chilly evening after receiving a report of a half-undressed man running in and out of busy traffic, barely missing being hit by speeding automobiles. He is a well-known individual named Sam who has been in many neighborhood group homes, but he often leaves without apparent reason, resulting in prolonged periods of homelessness. The man is brandishing a large tree branch and screaming at the cars as they pass. When police first contact Sam, he yells at them, "Shoot me now! Shoot me now!" He then wields the branch at them in a fighting pose. Police are able to coax him into putting down the branch and coming with them. While traveling in the squad car, Sam speaks very rapidly, sometimes unintelligibly, and repeatedly tells the police that the FBI and the president are plotting to kill him, so maybe he will kill himself first. Police place Sam on an involuntary psychiatric hold and transport him for treatment to a psychiatric emergency service (PES).

UTILIZATION OF PSYCHIATRIC EMERGENCY SERVICES BY THE MENTALLY ILL HOMELESS

Homeless individuals can reach a perilous level of psychiatric impairment in which they become too acutely ill to treat in a community setting. At this point, the PES plays an essential role in assessment, treatment, stabilization, and eventual referral for longer-term care. Statistically, the homeless mentally ill are high-frequency users of emergency systems (D'Amore et al. 2001). A study of visits to the PES in San Francisco showed that although homeless individuals constituted only 8% of the total mental health caseload for the city, they comprised one-third of emergency psychiatric visits. It was also noted in this study that homeless individuals were three times more likely to be treated in an emergency psychiatric setting after a violent episode than domiciled mental health clients. Homeless people were also more likely to be hospitalized from the episode and to have return emergency visits (McNiel and Binder 2005).

There is significant overlap between factors associated with homelessness and factors associated with repeat presentations to a PES (Pasic et al. 2005). On examination, Sam was found to have present many factors associated with high utilization of the PES, including homelessness, psychotic disorder, cocaine abuse, and lack of social supports (McNiel and Binder 2005). He was nonadherent to outpatient treatment and medication, lived in a state of poverty, and had medical comorbidities including diabetes and a history of hyperthyroidism. However, he was enrolled in Medicaid and intensive outpatient case management.

He is representative of the severely and persistently mentally ill group that frequently has benefits, more intensive outpatient treatment, and supportive housing or group home living arrangements, but who intermittently become noncompliant. In this group, illness exacerbation is swift and precipitous despite such supports, frequently necessitating hospitalization or provoking incarceration (Kuno et al. 2000). There is a second group of homeless individuals using the PES who are likely to have recently lost a job or spent money on drugs or alcohol instead of on rent. Personality disorders are common in this group. Borderline personality disorder presents with parasuicidal behaviors clustered around a recent loss. Antisocial personality disorder presents with evidence of malingering; a good example is the use of contingent suicide ("I'll kill myself if you don't admit me") to get food and shelter.

EMERGENCY PSYCHIATRIC TREATMENT OF THE MENTALLY ILL HOMELESS

The symptoms of homeless individuals such as Sam may be psychiatric in nature, a result of medical infirmity, or a combination of the two. Therefore, all patients with evidence of acute mental illness presenting to a PES are given an initial medical screening examination, including vital signs measurement (Allen et al. 2005a). After an initial screening by nursing personnel and the psychiatrist on duty, Sam was believed to be medically stable and in need of psychiatric diagnosis and treatment. Figure 8–1 illustrates the triage process for psychiatric emergency services.

Foremost in the PES evaluation is a determination of dangerousness to self and others. These are the predominant criteria used to permit involun-

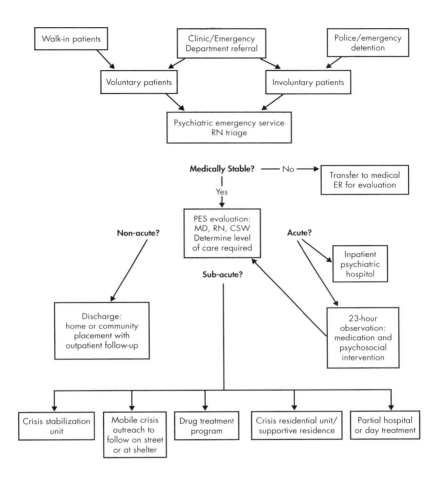

FIGURE 8–1. Flowchart of treatment: psychiatric emergency services (PES) for homeless persons.

CSW=certified social worker; ER=emergency room; RN=registered nurse.

tary psychiatric care (although many areas also permit detention based on *grave disability,* in which a person is so mentally impaired as to be unable to care for his or her own food, clothing, and shelter). A patient who is dangerous or gravely disabled may be treated against his or her will; if not, and if the patient wishes to leave, in most municipalities he or she must be released. In Sam's case, he demonstrated a danger to self in that he had asked police to kill him and a danger to others through threats of assault. He was also gravely disabled in that he was barely dressed and refusing to remain in his home on a cold night. Though demanding to leave the PES, he clearly met involuntary hold criteria, and so evaluation and treatment could proceed.

The evaluation reveals that Sam is still paranoid, fearful that that the FBI is after him. He is highly pressured, he is hyperactive, and he wants to hurt others and himself. He acknowledges smoking cocaine earlier in the day as well. After this evaluation and a review of his old records, he has a urine toxicology screen with positive results. Sam receives diagnoses of schizoaffective disorder, manic; and cocaine intoxication.

He is offered antipsychotic and sedative medications that he takes by mouth. Not long afterward, he is resting quietly in his room. In the morning, Sam wakes up dramatically improved. He is pleasant and cooperative, conversing logically at a normal rate, and is no longer paranoid or delusional. He has no thoughts of wanting to hurt others or himself and appears to have completely detoxified from the cocaine, and his acute psychiatric condition has stabilized. The psychiatrist and psychiatric resident who evaluate him agree that he should be able to be discharged and summon social services for assistance in disposition. Had Sam not improved so quickly, psychiatric inpatient hospitalization might have been considered.

A social worker and a social work intern meet with Sam. They discuss his difficulty with staying in the same residence. He reports that his last placement had easy access to drug dealers and that this offered too much temptation for him to not take medicine and instead use cocaine. On this basis, the team decides that temporary psychiatric housing with a focus on drug treatment may be an excellent opportunity and arranges placement in such a program for him in concert with his outpatient case manager. An appointment is made with his case management team and psychiatrist to see him after discharge.

This was a fortunate outcome. Obtaining follow-up medical care and case management helps to decrease future psychiatric emergencies (Clarke et al. 2000). Individuals who did not have an outpatient appointment after discharge have been shown to be two times more likely to be rehospitalized in the same year than those who kept at least one outpatient appointment (Nelson et al. 2000). But frequently, discharge planning for homeless individuals from the PES can be an arduous task. Chemical dependency treatment and housing, especially, can be difficult to obtain on brief notice.

With patients needing placement at all hours, even in the middle of the night, a shelter is the most likely short-term solution. But shelters are often reluctant to take referrals from a psychiatric facility. Stigma and misunderstanding of psychiatric illness can frighten shelter staff, and they may thus deny referrals from PES staff. Meanwhile, many chemical-dependency treatment programs feel their best chance for success is with motivated, sober individuals who have demonstrated over time the desire to get treatment. That such criteria are met can be exceptionally difficult to prove with homeless patients with co-occurring chemical dependency and mental illness in the PES. Those centers that do provide both housing and substance abuse interventions on an impromptu basis are unfortunately few in number. Twelve-step and faith-based programs are frequently ineffective in this population, and disaffection with such programs may become a deterrent to seeking further treatment for a co-occurring substance use disorder.

BUILDING RELATIONSHIPS WITH THE HOMELESS MENTALLY ILL IN THE PSYCHIATRIC EMERGENCY SERVICE

Coercion is defined as the use of force or threats to make people do things against their will, or the force used for this purpose. Unfortunately, the life of a homeless person with severe mental illness is often filled with an endless variety of coercive interactions. This often speaks to the inadequacy of the mental health system. For instance, some outreach workers and law enforcement officers might tell a mentally ill homeless person in distress that they are just taking him or her to the PES for medication and not for hospital admission, even though they know the person will likely require hospitalization. This deception and coercion is in great part a product of inadequate mobile acute care resources. Chapter 11 discusses how mobile crisis teams may be used to assist mentally ill homeless persons.

Also, many communities are using crisis intervention teams (CIT) to divert people from the criminal justice system (Steadman et al. 2000). CIT programs, first developed in Memphis, Tennessee, in 1988, are unique partnerships between police officers, mental health consumers and family members, local advocacy, university medical schools, and psychiatric emergency services. CITs are made up of volunteer police officers, who usually undergo 40 hours of coursework in how to quickly recognize and engage emotionally disturbed persons. CIT has been shown to positively affect officers' perceptions of mentally ill people, decrease the need for higher levels of police intervention (i.e., SWAT), decrease officer and patient injuries through less use of force and more use of verbal de-escalation, and redirect those in crisis from the criminal justice system to the health care system (Dupont and Cochran 2000).

When the police do bring a person to the PES, officers and mental health professionals heavily collaborate, pooling their combined knowledge of the patient and educating each other whenever possible. Officers provide historical information to PES staff about the community life and behaviors of the individual, and PES staff may formally and informally educate the police officers regarding mental status, diagnosis, substance use, and suicide/homicide risk assessment. PES staff works to ensure that the officers can return to their patrols as quickly as possible after the encounter, sometimes in 15 minutes or less. It is critical that both officers and mental health staff understand and respect each other's policies and procedures in the performance of their respective duties to ensure optimal and responsive care for the patient in crisis.

Unduly coercive behaviors can destroy the therapeutic alliance with the homeless patient. It is well known that in working with violent patients in the PES, the rapid formation of a therapeutic alliance will greatly decrease the likelihood of violence toward staff or other patients in the emergency room and the inpatient service (Beauford et al. 1997). If the PES visit is the patient's very first contact with the mental health care system, avoiding coercion can have a halo effect for many years to come. In our experience, this can profoundly increase the likelihood of subsequent adherence with outpatient treatment and medication.

So, how does one avoid coercion and develop this therapeutic relationship in the sterile, restrictive, chaotic environment that is the PES (Segal et al. 2001)? First, the PES applies the concept of *procedural justice,* in which the patient in crisis believes that he or she is meaningfully involved in the decision-making process and that the process is fair. In the PES, Sam was continuously engaged in a collaborative interaction, not a one-sided attempt to complete an assessment. The emergency psychiatrist on duty worked to elicit his wants; he was given the opportunity to speak without interruption, even though he was loud and hyperverbal. The assessment was accomplished taking into account decreased cognitive functioning. The staff prominently displayed empathy with and understanding of Sam's inner world.

Second, the staff worked with a goal of using the least restrictive intervention possible. The more restrictive a crisis intervention, the more coerced and victimized the homeless mentally ill patient may feel. Involuntary commitment should be used as a last resort with this population. It is now the standard of care to avoid, whenever possible, the use of seclusion, restraint, and medication over objection in the PES (Allen et al. 2005a). Avoiding these restrictive interventions reduces injuries to staff and patient, decreases stigma, and minimizes the harmful effects of coercion. When Sam initially presented to the PES, he was loud, threatening, and menacing. The PES staff intervened by asking the patient what he needed in order to calm down and by offering time out. They respected the patient's personal space, listened intently, avoided provocative language, established the desire to keep him safe, used simple language, and identified the patient's wants and needs. Verbal de-escalation creates a trust that is destroyed if one relies solely on seclusion or restraint (Allen et al. 2005b).

Third, PES staff should have the capacity to offer an array of less restrictive alternatives to hospitalization. Doing so enhances the therapeutic relationship by offering choice and the option of community-based treatment. What are these less restrictive alternatives? Patients may initially be placed in what is commonly referred to in our community as a *23-hour observation* for initial stabilization. Next, they might be offered a choice of three programs: 1) follow-up by the use of mobile psychiatric emergency teams, which send psychiatrists, nurses, and social workers to follow up with the individual, regardless of setting or location; 2) a crisis stabilization unit, a short-term treatment in a voluntary setting where psychiatrists makes daily rounds (this milieu is less restrictive and crowded than a typical inpatient psychiatric unit, and thus often appeals to homeless persons used to being on the streets); and 3) a crisis residential unit. This is a home in the community in which the person stays for several weeks, with nursing and social work oversight (Fenton et al. 2002). The milieu is kept minimally structured to encourage the homeless patient to want to come off the street and remain domiciled.

Patients often complain of arriving at the PES feeling angry, terrified, or demoralized. This can be reversed, leaving them with a sense of restored dignity, feeling calm and unafraid, or with a sense that things will improve for them (McNeil and Binder 2005). In our case study, Sam felt that his strengths, not his pathology, were emphasized. He especially noted the acts of kindness, including being given a blanket and being listened to respectfully. He expressed great appreciation for our not having used injections to calm him down.

CONCLUSION

Emergency psychiatrists often say that the PES is a barometer of the overall wellness of the local mental health care delivery system and of society's current values. The patients coming to the PES reflect society's understandings or misunderstandings concerning mental illness, as well as the level to which a community has committed to diversion from jail and to less restrictive community alternatives to hospitalization. The PES continues to be widely used by the uninsured, the undocumented, and those on waiting lists for outpatient slots (Wu and Serper 1999). Concerning aiding homeless people, the psychiatric emergency service can provide attractive alternatives to the hospital or jail.

REFERENCES

Allen MH, Currier GW, Carpenter D, et al: Treatment of behavioral emergencies 2005. J Psychiatr Pract 11 (suppl 1):5–108, 2005a

Allen MH, Carpenter D, Sheets JL, et al: What do consumers say they want and need during a psychiatric emergency? J Psychiatr Pract 9:39–58, 2005b

Beauford JE, McNiel DE, Binder RL: Utility of the initial therapeutic alliance in evaluating psychiatric patients' risk of violence. Am J Psychiatry 154:1272–1276, 1997

Clarke GN, Herinckx HA, Kinney RF, et al: Psychiatric hospitalizations, arrests, emergency room visits, and homelessness of clients with serious and persistent mental illness: findings from a randomized trial of two ACT programs vs. usual care. Ment Health Serv Res 2:155–164, 2000

D'Amore J, Hung O, Chiang W, et al: The epidemiology of the homeless population and its impact on an urban emergency department. Acad Emerg Med 8:1051–1055, 2001

Dupont R, Cochran S: Police response to mental health emergencies—barriers to change. J Am Acad Psychiatry Law 28:338–344, 2000

Fenton WS, Hoch JS, Herrell JM, et al: Cost and cost-effectiveness of hospital vs. residential crisis care for patients who have serious mental illness. Arch Gen Psychiatry 59:357–364, 2002

Kuno E, Rothbard AB, Averyt J, et al: Homelessness among persons with serious mental illness in an enhanced community-based mental health system. Psychiatr Serv 51:1012–1016, 2000

McNiel DE, Binder RL: Psychiatric emergency service use and homelessness, mental disorder, and violence. Psychiatr Serv 56:699–704, 2005

Nelson EA, Maruish ME, Axler JL: Effects of discharge planning and compliance with outpatient appointments on readmission rates. Psychiatr Serv 51:885–889, 2000

Pasic J, Russo J, Roy-Byrne P: High utilizers of psychiatric emergency services. Psychiatr Serv 56:678–684, 2005

Segal SP, Laurie TA, Segal MJ: Factors in the use of coercive retention in civil commitment evaluations in psychiatric emergency services. Psychiatr Serv 52:514–520, 2001

Steadman HJ, Deane MW, Borum R, et al: Comparing outcomes of major models of police responses to mental health emergencies. Psychiatr Serv 51:645–649, 2000

Wu T, Serper MR: Social support and psychopathology in homeless patients presenting for emergency psychiatric treatment. J Clin Psychol 55:1127–1133, 1999

Chapter 9

PSYCHIATRIC INPATIENT SETTINGS

David Nardacci, M.D.

John is a single 38-year-old man with chronic undifferentiated schizophrenia who has a 15-year history of homelessness. He shunned the city shelter system, preferring to stay in a busy public transportation hub where he would sit along the wall passively, sometimes accepting handouts from passersby, sometimes rummaging through garbage cans to find food. His behavior never escalated toward violence, and his negligence in self-care never progressed to the point of requiring involuntary hospitalization. It wasn't until he began masturbating in public that he captured the attention of the transit police, who brought him to a hospital emergency department.

John was hospitalized on New York's first homeless inpatient unit at Bellevue Hospital, where he received intensive specialized care that was ultimately successful. He had many of the common medical problems that beset homeless people living in public areas: he was lice infested, underweight, and anemic, with a folate deficiency. He also had a positive result on the PPD skin test for tuberculosis.

John initially refused all medications and was taken to court so that he could be given medication over objection. He began a course of haloperidol decanoate and gradually improved over a period of several weeks. He continued to display prominent negative symptomatology but began showing improvements in self-care, and his verbalizations increased. Although his level of insight was only marginally improved, he did accept oral benztropine and received injections without overt resistance.

With persistence and frequent nonthreatening contact, staff gradually gained his confidence and were able to obtain sufficient information to contact his long-lost family on the West Coast. To the staff's amazement, John actually had a master's degree in engineering and had held a relatively high-paying job in his mid-twenties. However, as his illness emerged he was no longer able to sustain employment and within 2 years he began a lengthy period of homelessness. He had two brief hospitalizations early in the course of his illness but was discharged without firm housing plans and returned almost immediately to homelessness, wandering across the country and ending up in New York City.

On the homeless unit, he had a 2-month stay that allowed staff sufficient time to find an attractive placement site able to provide the necessary level of supervision that John required. Staff took special care to elicit his responses to each of the potential housing sites, incorporating his preferences in the final selection process. A housing provider with 24-hour staffing that provided meals and on-site case management services was eventually chosen. John was also referred to a day treatment program for additional rehabilitation. He was discharged on haloperidol decanoate 100 mg once every 4 weeks and benztropine 1 mg twice daily with minimal evidence of extrapyramidal side effects.

Follow-up inquiries indicated that John was still housed at 3 months, 6 months, and 1 year and had not required rehospitalization. He made further modest gains in his level of functioning and was considering transfer to a less supervised type of housing.

INPATIENT ASSESSMENT

The initial foundation for therapeutic success is comprehensive biopsychosocial assessment by a coordinated team with multiple areas of expertise.

Getting the Diagnosis Right

One of the commonest reasons for system failure in the rehabilitation of mentally ill homeless people is the failure to make a fully accurate psychiatric assessment at the time of inpatient hospitalization. Common problems include the following:

- Failure to elicit subtle psychotic symptomatology
- Misdiagnosis of substance-abusing patients with "personality disorders" when there is actually major Axis I pathology present
- Failure to identify comorbid substance abuse in more regressed psychotic patients
- Failure to recognize bipolarity and mood symptoms
- Inadequate screening for cognitive impairments
- Failure to elicit past abuse/trauma history and recognize trauma-related symptomatology
- Failure to perform a nonadherence risk assessment

Eliciting Subtle Psychotic Symptoms

Even the casual passerby can recognize a floridly psychotic individual like John who appears grossly disheveled and disorganized, obviously responding to internal stimuli. For the vast majority of homeless individuals, however, the signs of psychosis are considerably more subtle, and it is quite common for patients to exhibit profound levels of denial that are at least partially related to the underlying cognitive dysfunction of the illness itself (Amador et al. 1994; Weickert et al. 2000). It is important that clinicians not automatically accept this initial denial at face value and that they probe carefully for auditory hallucinations and covert delusional ideation with additional questions.

Looking Beyond Obvious "Substance Abuse"

There is a substantially increased incidence of alcohol and substance abuse among mentally ill homeless people, and substance abuse is clearly one of the biggest risk factors associated with repeat homelessness (Drake et al. 1993; Folsom et al. 2005; Koegel et al. 1988). Some homeless individuals come into contact with the mental health system only after they have created a public disturbance while in an intoxicated state, and many of these individuals have histories of recurrent brief hospitalizations. Once a primary substance use disorder has become of part of the patient's hospital record, clinicians who subsequently review the patient's record may fail to perform a careful diagnostic evaluation. Disorganized thinking or mood lability are written off in error as intoxication related. The patients are eager for discharge and will deny or minimize symptomatology, and hospital-based clinicians will readily oblige these "difficult" patients by discharging them prematurely (Drake et al. 1966).

Identifying Covert Substance Abuse

The converse problem also exists, especially the failure of clinicians to recognize substance abuse problems in patients with primarily negative symptomatology. A large community survey (Mueser et al. 2004) indicated that even among homeless individuals with chronic undifferentiated schizophrenia, rates of alcohol and substance abuse were increased by 240%. Alcohol or substance misuse is often the critical factor precipitating the homelessness of an otherwise marginally compensated individual (Schutt et al. 1996).

Recognizing Mood Disorders

Another common diagnostic error is the failure of many clinicians to accurately diagnose and treat the mood components of illness. Patients have been erroneously given diagnoses of primary substance abuse, borderline personality, or schizophrenia, or given no diagnosis at all. Marked irritability/lability or motor agitation in a patient who is not acutely intoxicated is highly suggestive of a mood disorder. Bipolar disorders may be difficult to diagnose accurately without a reliable past history or reliable collateral information (Akiskal and Pinto 1999; Escamilla 2001). Underdiagnosis of bipolar disorder is particularly common with African American patients (Strakowski et al. 2003).

Screening for Cognitive Deficits

As a group, mentally ill homeless individuals have more severe cognitive impairments than their non-homeless counterparts (Solliday-McRoy et al. 2004). They are more likely to have comorbid mental retardation, focal brain injuries, or medically related amnestic disorders and dementias. On the Bellevue homeless inpatient unit, 45% of 73 patients identified as having significant cognitive deficits on the basis of routine mental status exams had abnormal computed tomographic (CT) scans—most commonly showing nonspecific cerebral atrophy—and 26% had abnormal electroencephalograms (Nardacci et al. 1993).

Identifying Trauma-Related Symptoms

Familial disintegration is clearly one of many core factors that have contributed to the current homeless crisis (Koegel et al. 1995; Susser et al. 1991). Many mentally ill homeless persons have come from highly dysfunctional families, often with at least one mentally ill parent, and many have passed through the foster care system as children (Susser et al. 1991). Multiple case studies have shown increased rates of early neglect and abuse among the homeless and they are more likely to have trauma-related syndromes such as posttraumatic stress disorder and dissociative disorders (Mueser et al. 2004).

Performing a Nonadherence Risk Assessment

No psychiatric assessment of a homeless person with mental illness would be complete without a careful assessment of past nonadherence. Treatment nonadherence is multifactorial but usually involves a significant element of denial. Denial can be a normative reaction to any serious illness; however, in persons with severe mental illness it is also influenced by neurologically based cognitive and perceptual distortions intrinsic to the underlying illness (Ruscher et al. 1997; Stoudemire and Thompson 1983). In some instances, nonadherence occurs as a byproduct of negative experiences with the health delivery system and/or medication side effects (Ruscher et al. 1997; Stoudemire and Thompson 1983). Not infrequently, past substance abuse has been a major contributing factor. It is important to realize, however, that treatment nonadherence can also be approached as a manifestation of the healthy desire for autonomy and often occurs in the context of symptom resolution and an increasing sense of normalcy (Stoudemire and Thompson 1983).

Inpatient Medical Assessment

Without question, one of the greatest assets of the inpatient setting is the ready access to a wide range of diagnostic and treatment resources. Patients can receive complex diagnostic workups within days and have immediate access to specialty medical consultations. Tuberculosis is of particular concern, and there is a growing awareness of hepatitis C and HIV infection in the homeless population. Homeless individuals are susceptible to the same major medical illnesses that afflict the general population, but they are likely to have gone for extended periods either undiagnosed or untreated, leading to secondary organ damage (Breakey et al. 1989; Empfield et al. 1993; Sherriff et al. 2003).

The inpatient medical assessment of the mentally ill homeless individual should include a complete blood count with differential, a complete metabolic panel including lipids, thyroid function tests, and screening tests for hepatitis and syphilis. HIV testing should be strongly considered for those in higher risk categories and included in any inpatient neurological workup (Nardacci et al. 1993).

Tuberculosis skin testing should be performed routinely on homeless individuals with unknown status, and positive skin test results require vigorous follow-up including chest X-rays and sputum testing if indicated. Patients with demonstrable cognitive deficits warrant cerebral scanning procedures, with noncontrast CT scanning as an absolute minimum (Nardacci et al. 1993). Patients phobic about tests like magnetic resonance imaging and CT scans can be accompanied by supportive staff and premedicated with 1–2 mg of oral or intramuscular lorazepam.

Inpatient Psychosocial Assessment

Obtaining useful psychosocial data on homeless individuals often requires a high level of persistence and ingenuity on the part of the hospital staff. A good hospital assessment should include a meticulous housing and entitlements history along with a comprehensive search for collateral information from the patient's social support network, community treatment providers, and past treatment settings. It is especially important to know whether the patient has been placed in supportive settings before and what factors may have contributed to the patient's "falling out" of housing. In many hospitals, the comprehensive psychosocial assessment is typically performed just after admission. With regressed, chronically psychotic individuals, particularly those with depression or negative schizophrenic symptoms however, it is often more appropriate to wait several weeks until medication has begun working and the patient has engaged with staff (Golub et al. 1993).

INPATIENT HOSPITALIZATION: A WINDOW OF OPPORTUNITY

The inpatient stay offers a unique opportunity to initiate complex treatment strategies that may be unavailable in other treatment settings. Some of these include:

- Participation in a structured therapeutic milieu
- Access to state-of-the-art pharmacological interventions
- Reliable administration of medication
- Access to court-ordered interventions

> John derived clear benefit from the concentrated resources available in an in-patient setting. His nutritional deficiencies were rapidly identified and corrected. He was started on a haloperidol decanoate preparation that would be practical postdischarge. With the combined benefits of medication and the inpatient therapeutic milieu, he was able to disclose personal information that enabled staff to locate his family of origin.

The Therapeutic Milieu

Hospital-based psychoeducation and medication teaching improve postdischarge treatment outcome (Henry and Ghaemi 2004; Stoudemire and Thompson 1983). Hospital staff can reinforce adherence by offering patients prompt accurate here-and-now feedback as they observe subtle changes in the patient's day-to-day functioning. Pointing out to the patient that he or she is sleeping, grooming, socializing, or concentrating better strengthens the therapeutic alliance and reinforces the value of the treatment.

Structured therapeutic activities on an inpatient unit can have a powerful therapeutic effect. They offer a safe, nonthreatening venue for self-expression and socialization without invoking the anxiety of more direct forms of self-disclosure. For more verbal and socially adept patients, drama therapies with assigned role-playing can be highly beneficial. Acting out guided "street scenes" on the Bellevue inpatient unit created an opportunity for patients to receive approval and affirmation from their peers, allowing them to feel more connected and less like unwanted "outsiders" (Golub et al. 1993). Seemingly withdrawn, socially awkward patients will sometimes engage surprisingly well through nonverbal music and art therapies. Even the most psychotic patients still retain some ability to communicate individual thoughts and feelings through the creative process, and many homeless individuals with chronic psychosis show striking originality in their artwork.

Positive inpatient group experiences facilitate the transition to outpatient day treatment settings, laying the groundwork for future participation in groups where more extensive psychosocial rehabilitation can occur.

Proactive Psychopharmacological Interventions

Mentally ill homeless people require a substantial reduction of symptoms in order to make a successful transition after discharge. A 50% reduction in psychotic symptoms, which might be regarded as an acceptable treatment outcome for a patient with solid community supports, may be woefully inadequate for a disaffiliated person with protracted homelessness. To achieve the requisite level of response, the patient may require multiple medication trials and/or combination therapies. It is unusual for a patient to achieve the desired level of functioning with just one trial of a single agent (Levy 1993; Zarate and Quinoz 2003).

Combinations of antipsychotics and mood-stabilizing agents are often indicated, and many patients with neuroleptic-refractory symptoms warrant trials of clozapine (Levy 1993; Reus 1993; Zarate and Quiroz 2003). These complex trials may be difficult to conduct on an outpatient basis. The inpatient setting offers ready access to blood work and frequent monitoring of vital signs, enabling rapid medication titration. Side effects can be detected more quickly, lessening patient discomfort and reducing the likelihood of serious complications. The inpatient setting is also an ideal place to make proactive medication choices that will decrease long-term health risks such as obesity and the "metabolic syndrome" (Faulkner et al. 2003).

In-House Medication Monitoring

Covert medication nonadherence is commonplace, even in hospital settings, and accounts for a high percentage of supposed "treatment failures" (Henry and Ghaemi 2004). Hospital-based nursing staff may be more adept at detecting "cheeking" and other forms of covert nonadherence and have ready access to liquids and short-acting injectables unavailable in other settings. Careful medication administration and monitoring in the hospital setting ensures maximal benefit from the medication and enables the psychiatrist to make subsequent medication decisions more accurately.

Court-Mandated Interventions

Patients who perpetually refuse to take psychotropic medications are overrepresented among the mentally ill homeless. Even patients able to sustain contact with community social service providers often remain "locked out" of housing options on the basis of their refusal to accept medication. Successful physician-initiated requests for medication over objection can be life-changing and reverse years of therapeutic stalemate for some of these patients.

Although there is wide variation in municipal and state laws, most states offer the possibility of medication over objection, and many now allow for involuntary administration of medication to outpatients as well (Torrey and Zdanowicz 2001). The importance of these interventions cannot be overemphasized, particularly for patients who have had repeated hospitalizations for nonadherence. Court-mandated interventions buy additional time for the patient to develop critical insight into the benefits of treatment. Court-mandated interventions can also be used to obtain in-hospital medical testing over objection, to arrange for guardianship, or to structure required postdischarge treatment services (Patel and Hardy 2001; Sabatini et al. 1993).

Developing an Inpatient Treatment Plan

Effective treatment planning for the mentally ill homeless incorporates short-term institutionally based goals into a more comprehensive long-term vision, creating a therapeutic framework that will facilitate successful community transition and sustained wellness. Elements critical to success include:

- Building a meaningful therapeutic alliance and creating therapeutic momentum that can be carried beyond discharge
- Establishing a viable long-term medication regime, utilizing court-ordered interventions when necessary
- Extending length of stay sufficiently to secure a substantive improvement in symptoms
- Meticulous attention to the process of aftercare referral and housing placement

> John's inpatient treatment plan was clearly instrumental in laying the groundwork for his postdischarge success. He was given appropriate medication and hospitalized for a sufficient length of time to achieve clinically significant improvement in his level of functioning. Although he remained moderately symptomatic, he had successfully established a therapeutic alliance with the treatment team and was actively engaged in his own discharge planning process.

Therapeutic Engagement

Many homeless individuals have lost the support of familial relationships and "community" (Golub et al. 1993; Lehman et al. 1995; Sullivan et al. 2000). Many women have lost custody of their children and suffer persistent feelings of anger and loss (Mullick et al. 2001). For some individuals the chaotic world of auditory hallucinations and delusions actually serves a defensive function, offering a sense of importance and of connection with an otherwise hurtful and rejecting world. Successful therapeutic work with these patients must include some acknowledgment of loss and must confront the powerful effects of stigma in order to establish a viable therapeutic alliance and begin the corrective process of rebuilding fragile self-esteem (Cohen 1989; Golub et al. 1993; Huszonek 1987).

Length of Stay Considerations

The current mandate of most inpatient facilities is to move patients through the hospital rapidly. The goal is to contain symptoms rather than provide rehabilitation, an approach that is often antithetical to long-range success with the chronically homeless.

The typical patient with a history of prolonged homelessness and treatment recidivism will require a minimum of several weeks in the hospital. The standard discharge criterion of no longer posing an imminent "danger to self or others" is likely to result in premature discharge with a high likelihood of relapse and a rapid return to homelessness (Dion et al. 1988; Goldfinger et al. 1996; Kertesz et al. 2003).The patient should improve to the extent that positive psychotic symptoms and any associated manic or mixed mood symptoms no longer drive the patient's day-to-day behaviors. By the time of discharge, the patient needs to be well engaged in treatment and disposition planning, voicing genuine acceptance of the proposed aftercare plan.

Some chronic mentally ill homeless persons actually need transfer to longer-term treatment facilities that can provide sufficient time for clinically meaningful change to occur. Securing additional treatment time at one of these facilities can mean the difference between success and failure with the most severely ill subgroup of patients and is well worth advocating for (Schrage et al. 1993; Sood et al. 1996).

COMMUNITY PLACEMENT

Securing Entitlements

Applications for Supplemental Security Income or Social Security Disability Insurance benefits should be initiated promptly while the patient is still in an inpatient setting and warrants meticulous documentation. Recounting past symptoms may be insufficient; the degree of current and projected disability must be convincingly stated. The application should offer specific details about the patient's current functioning and offer concrete reasons why the patient cannot be gainfully employed in the immediate future even if receiving appropriate treatment. Emphasizing the nature and extent of the patient's recent homelessness is important, and stressing the patient's need for placement in supportive housing lends additional weight.

Patients with histories of substance abuse are particularly vulnerable to rejection unless a psychiatric disability apart from the substance abuse has been clearly defined. Patients who go to the Social Security office on their own without independent documentation are also more likely to be rejected, and an appeal can take as long as 18 months. Rejected applications often result from misdiagnosis. Many homeless individuals given a diagnosis of "depression" on their original disability applications actually have unrecognized bipolar mood disorders or schizophrenia. If a patient was misdiagnosed and the denial of benefits was recent, it is more advantageous to initiate a brand-new application with a modified diagnosis and better substantiating information.

When families or other representative payees have been receiving a homeless mentally ill person's disability checks, it is important for inpatient staff to intervene on the patient's behalf and reroute this money so the patient can begin purchasing essential items and have the necessary funds to secure supportive housing.

Primacy of Aftercare Planning

The homeless patient is most vulnerable during the immediate postdischarge period, and choosing appropriate postdischarge treatment modalities is critical (Goldfinger et al. 1996; Kertesz et al. 2003). Patients with histories of repeated treatment failure and nonadherence need higher levels of treatment structure. Even for individuals placed in well-supervised housing sites, traditional clinic treatment is not likely to be sufficient (Bustillo et al. 2001). Strong consideration should be given to more intensive interventions, including:

- Continuing day treatment (including programs for co-occurring chemical dependency)
- Partial hospitalization programs
- Assertive Community Treatment (ACT)
- Court-mandated outpatient treatment
- Case management services

Day treatment programs offer the opportunity for ongoing psychosocial rehabilitation. Effective programs promote psychoeducation, socialization, activities of daily living skills enhancement, creative self-expression, and vocational readiness. The partial hospitalization program provides a more intensively structured milieu that may be necessary for patients who have had briefer inpatient stays with substantial residual symptomatology at the time of discharge (Horvitz-Lennon et al. 2001). Postdischarge substance abuse is highly correlated with treatment failure and repeat homelessness, and discharge planning must factor in the need for dual treatment and perhaps for more restrictive residential treatment in some cases (Gonzalez and Rosenheck 2002).

Without question, many homeless mentally ill individuals are best served by ACT teams and/or court-mandated outpatient commitment, and there is a strong evidence base supporting both of these practices. These types of services are often more difficult to access from outpatient settings and are best secured while the patient is still hospitalized. Having ACT or mandated outpatient treatment in place can be especially valuable during the high-risk period immediately after discharge (Dixon et al. 1997).

Case management services are also acknowledged as valuable adjuncts to the overall treatment package of patients with histories of poor therapeutic engagement and repeated hospitalization.

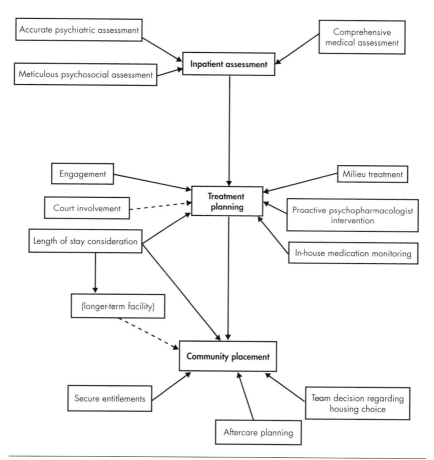

FIGURE 9–1. Key elements of inpatient psychiatric treatment.

Key elements in the inpatient assessment, treatment, and community placement process are summarized in Figure 9–1.

The Challenge of Housing Choice

Chronically homeless individuals generally underestimate the amount of community assistance they are likely to require (Barrow et al. 1989; Goldfinger et al. 1996; Schutt and Goldfinger 1996); hospitals, on the other hand, tend to underestimate nonadherence risk and to select housing sites with inadequate levels of supervision (Barrow et al. 1989; Goering et al. 1984; Goldfinger et al. 1999; Owen et al. 1997).

The responsibility for placement decisions often devolves entirely onto the inpatient social work staff, but is better served by input from the entire inpatient treatment team. Psychiatrists' specialized assessment skills actually make them ideally qualified to evaluate patients' treatment motivation and nonadherence risk, yet they often remain peripheral to important placement and aftercare decisions being made.

It is equally important to actively involve the patient's existing support network and community caregivers in the discharge planning process, making full use of their past experience with the client (Hurlburt et al. 1996; Owen et al. 1997; Srebnik et al. 1998) in order to avoid repeating past errors and perpetuating the cycle of homelessness.

The housing selection process dramatizes the fundamental therapeutic challenge facing psychiatric inpatient units at the present time; namely, the challenge of accepting greater ownership of their potential role within the larger service continuum. There is a clear opportunity for inpatient units to assume greater responsibility for the long-range treatment planning of each homeless person they serve, working in concert with other providers to restore a lasting sense of "home" and "community" through personal empowerment.

REFERENCES

Akiskal H, Pinto O: The evolving bipolar spectrum: prototypes I, II, III, and IV. Psychiatr Clin North Am 22:517–534, 1999

Amador X, Flaum M, Andreasen N, et al: Awareness of illness in schizophrenia and schizoaffective and mood disorders. Arch Gen Psychiatry 51:826–836, 1994

Barrow S, Hellman F, Lovell A, et al: Effectiveness of Programs for the Mentally Ill Homeless: Final Report. New York, New York State Psychiatric Institute, 1989

Breakey W, Fischer P, Kramer M, et al: Health and mental health problems of homeless men and women in Baltimore. JAMA 262:1352–1357, 1989

Bustillo J, Lauriello J, Horan W, et al: The psychosocial treatment of schizophrenia: an update. Am J Psychiatry 158:163–175, 2001

Cohen MK: Social work practice with homeless mentally ill people: engaging the client. Soc Work 34:505–509, 1989

Dion GL, Tohen M, Anthony WA, et al: Symptoms and functioning of patients with bipolar disorder six months after hospitalization. Hosp Community Psychiatry 39:652–657, 1988

Dixon L, Weiden P, Torres M, et al: Assertive community treatment and medication compliance in the homeless mentally ill. Am J Psychiatry 154:1302–1304, 1997

Drake RE, Alterman AI, Rosenberg SR: Detection of substance abuse disorders in severely ill mental patients. Community Ment Health J 29:175–192, 1993

Drake RE, Mueser KT, Clark RE, et al: The course, treatment, and outcome of substance disorder in persons with severe mental illness. Am J Orthopsychiatry 66:41–52, 1966

Empfield M, Cournos F, Meyer I, et al: HIV seropositivity among homeless patients admitted to a psychiatric inpatient unit. Am J Psychiatry 150:47–52, 1993

Escamilla MA: Diagnosis and treatment of mood disorders that co-occur with schizophrenia. Psychiatr Serv 52:911–919, 2001

Faulkner G, Soundy A, Lloyd K: Schizophrenia and weight management: a systematic review of interventions to control weight. Acta Psychiatr Scand 108:324–332, 2003

Folsom D, Hawthorne W, Lindamer L, et al: Prevalence of risk factors for homelessness and utilization of mental health services among 10,340 patients with serious mental illness in a large public mental health system. Am J Psychiatry 162:370–376, 2005

Goering P, Wasylenki D, Lancee W, et al: From hospital to community: six-month and two-year outcomes for 505 patients. J Nerv Ment Dis 172:667–673, 1984

Goldfinger SM, Schutt RK, Turner W, et al: Assessing homeless mentally ill persons for permanent housing: screening for safety. Community Ment Health J 32:275–288, 1996

Goldfinger SM, Schutt RK, Tolomiczenko GS, et al. Housing placement and subsequent days homeless among formerly homeless adults with mental illness. Psychiatr Serv 50:674–679, 1999

Golub W, Nardacci D, Frohock J, et al: Interdisciplinary strategies for engagement and rehabilitation, in Intensive Treatment of the Homeless Mentally Ill. Edited by Katz S, Nardacci D, Sabatini A. Washington, DC, American Psychiatric Press, 1993, pp 107–128

Gonzalez G, Rosenheck RA: Outcomes and service use among homeless persons with serious mental illness and substance abuse. Psychiatr Serv 53:437–446, 2002

Henry C, Ghaemi SN: Insight in psychosis: a systematic review of treatment interventions. Psychopathology 37:194–199, 2004

Horvitz-Lennon M, Normand S, Gaccione P, et al: Partial versus full hospitalization for adults in psychiatric distress: a systematic review of the published literature (1957–1997). Am J Psychiatry 158:676–685, 2001

Hurlburt M, Wood P, Hough R: Providing independent housing for the homeless mentally ill: a novel approach to evaluating long-term longitudinal housing patterns. J Community Psychol 24:291–310, 1996

Huszonek JJ: Establishing therapeutic contact with schizophrenics: a supervisory approach. Am J Psychother 41: 185–193, 1987

Kertesz SG, Horton NJ, Friedmann PD, et al: Slowing the revolving door: stabilization programs reduce homeless persons' substance abuse after detoxification. J Subst Abuse Treat 24:197–207, 2003

Koegel P, Burnam MA, Farr RK: The prevalence of specific psychiatric disorders among homeless individuals in the inner city of Los Angeles. Arch Gen Psychiatry 45:1085–1092, 1988

Koegel P, Melamid E, Burnam M: Childhood risk factors for homelessness among homeless adults. Am J Public Health 85:1642–1649, 1995

Lehman AF, Kernan E, DeForge BR, et al: Effects of homelessness on the quality of life of persons with severe mental illness. Psychiatr Serv 46:922–926, 1995

Levy RH: Psychopharmacological interventions, in Intensive Treatment of the Homeless Mentally Ill. Edited by Katz S, Nardacci D, Sabatini A. Washington, DC, American Psychiatric Press, 1993, pp 129–165

Mueser KT, Salyers MP, Rosenberg SD, et al: Interpersonal trauma and posttraumatic stress disorder in patients with severe mental illness: demographic, clinical, and health correlates. Schizophr Bull 30:45–57, 2004

Mullick M, Miller LJ, Jacobsen T: Insight into mental illness and child maltreatment risk among mothers with major psychiatric disorders. Psychiatr Serv 52:488–492, 2001

Nardacci D, Caro Y, Milstein V, et al: Bellevue population: demographics, in Intensive Treatment of the Homeless Mentally Ill. Edited by Katz S, Nardacci D, Sabatini A. Washington, DC, American Psychiatric Press, 1993, pp 51–70

Owen C, Rutherford V, Jones M, et al: Noncompliance in psychiatric aftercare. Community Ment Health J 33:25–34, 1997

Patel M, Hardy DW: Encouraging pursuit of court-ordered treatment in a state hospital. Psychiatr Serv 52:1656–1657, 2001

Reus VI: Rational polypharmacy in the treatment of mood disorders. Ann Clin Psychiatry 5:91–100, 1993

Ruscher SM, de Wit R, Mazmanian D: Psychiatric patients' attitudes about medication and factors affecting noncompliance. Psychiatr Serv 48:82–85, 1997

Sabatini A, Nardacci D, Katz S: Future directions, in Intensive Treatment of the Homeless Mentally Ill. Edited by Katz S, Nardacci D, Sabatini A. Washington, DC, American Psychiatric Press, 1993, pp 129–165

Schrage H, Silver M, Oldham J: Role of the state mental health system, in Intensive Treatment of the Homeless Mentally Ill. Edited by Katz S, Nardacci D, Sabatini A. Washington, DC, American Psychiatric Press, 1993, pp 129–165

Schutt RK, Goldfinger SM: Housing preferences and perceptions of health functioning among homeless mentally ill persons. Psychiatr Serv 47:381–386, 1996

Sherriff LC, Mayon-White RT: A survey of hepatitis C prevalence among the homeless community of Oxford. J Public Health Med 25:358–361, 2003

Solliday-McRoy C, Campbell TC, Melchert TP: Neuropsychological functioning of homeless men. J Nerv Ment Dis 192:471–478, 2004

Sood S, Baker M, Bledin K: Social and living skills of new long-stay hospital patients and new long-term community patients. Psychiatr Serv 47:619–622, 1996

Srebnik D, Uehara E, Smukler M: Field test of tool for level-of-care decisions in community mental health systems. Psychiatr Serv 49:91–97, 1998

Stoudemire A, Thompson TL 2nd: Medication noncompliance: systematic approaches to evaluation and intervention. Gen Hosp Psychiatry 5:233–239, 1983

Strakowski SM, Keck PE Jr, Arnold LM, et al: Ethnicity and diagnosis in patients with affective disorders. J Clin Psychiatry 78:747–754, 2003

Sullivan G, Burnam A, Koegel P, et al: Quality of life of homeless persons with mental illness: results from the course-of-homelessness study. Psychiatr Serv 51:1135–1141, 2000

Susser ES, Lin SP, Conover SA, et al: Childhood antecedents of homelessness in psychiatric patients. Am J Psychiatry 148:1026–1030, 1991

Torrey E, Zdanowicz M: Outpatient commitment: what, why, and for whom. Psychiatr Serv 52:337–341, 2001

Weickert TW, Goldberg TE, Gold JM, et al: Cognitive impairments in patients with schizophrenia displaying preserved and compromised intellect. Arch Gen Psychiatry 57:907–913 [erratum: 47(12):122], 2000

Zarate CA Jr, Quiroz JA: Combination treatment in bipolar disorder: review of controlled trials. Bipolar Disord 5:217–225 [erratum: 5(4):307], 2003

Chapter 10

PRIMARY CARE SETTINGS

Brian D. Bronson, M.D.
Anne M. Piette, L.M.S.W.

M̲r. L is a 69-year-old man who came to the hospital medical walk-in clinic reporting that he was homeless. He said, "I need help." The triage nurse noted that he was "a poor historian without a clear reason for his visit."

Although Mr. L denied medical complaints, he was seen by Dr. K, who ordered routine lab tests and discovered that Mr. L had elevated serum glucose and hemoglobin A1C. He told Mr. L that he had new-onset diabetes and that he could pick up his medication later at the pharmacy. That evening, after finishing his clinical work, Dr. K submitted electronic consultations with the social work service and with the pharmacy service to obtain glucose-lowering medication. A month later, Mr. L presented again to the emergency department with similarly vague complaints. He had never picked up his diabetic medication, his serum glucose remained elevated, and he denied that he had diabetes or other medical problems. The emergency department physician felt that Mr. L had an anxiety disorder and referred him to the mental health clinic, where he was given a diagnosis of schizophrenia, residual type. However, Mr. L also denied having a psychiatric condition and declined psychopharmacologic treatment. He was unsuccessfully referred to the social work service, and no further attempts at outreach occurred. Mr. L was admitted to the hospital medical service several months later with an acute myocardial infarction.

INTEGRATED PRIMARY CARE CLINICS

A fundamental issue concerning psychiatric competency in primary care settings is that primary care staff generally have modest training in mental health diagnosis and treatment (Sullivan et al. 1996). Because referral to a mental health clinician in primary care depends largely on the ability of primary care staff to recognize the need for referral, there is often inadequate recognition of psychiatric illness in primary care settings. Recognizing this need,

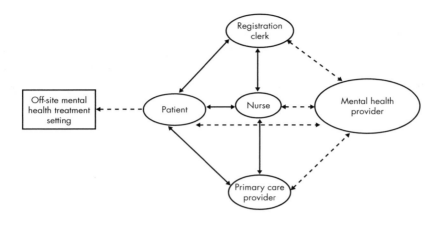

FIGURE 10–1.   Flowchart of treatment: primary care settings.

some primary care clinics have integrated staff with specialized mental health training into their clinical settings (Wedding and Mengel 2004). The extent of this integration is variable across clinics, both with respect to the specific mental health disciplines represented and the level of staffing. Although on-site mental health specialists may include one or more psychiatrists, psychologists, psychiatric nurse practitioners, or psychiatric social workers, often there is only a single mental health staff member, assigned on a full-time or part-time basis.

Figure 10–1 illustrates the flow of treatment for homeless patients in a primary care clinic with co-located mental health professionals. In some cases, the mental health provider is directly consulting with or treating a patient. In others, treatment occurs through "curbside consultation" and water-cooler case discussions with the primary care provider. Collaborative, multidisciplinary care is very important, especially because clinical engagement is often slow in this disaffiliated population and an individual's personal history may emerge over time and through a variety of channels. The mental health specialist in general, and the psychiatrist in particular, has a special role in guiding this clinical process. The mental health specialist in this setting may have an additional educational role in teaching other health professionals in primary care about medical interviewing and psychiatric evaluation and treatment of their patients.

MAKING THE DIAGNOSIS

Homeless patients in this setting often do not spontaneously report to primary care staff their psychiatric symptoms or a need for mental health intervention. Some patients, such as Mr. L, have psychotic denial of their medical or psychiatric illness. Others present with vague physical complaints, the repeated investigation of which does not lead to diagnosis of a primary underlying nonpsychiatric medical condition. Primary care patients with this presentation (sometimes referred to as *somatization*) often do not identify themselves as having a psychiatric need and therefore decline referral for mental health services. They may even be offended by suggestion that their symptoms are "all in their head." Other patients are hesitant to bother their busy primary care clinician with nonphysical complaints. For all of these reasons, many patients in primary care with psychiatric illness remain undiagnosed and therefore untreated.

To improve mental health case finding in primary care, mental health staff co-located in this setting should assume an active and collaborative role with primary care providers. The mental health clinician cannot work in isolation, but rather should be integrated into the routine operations of the particular primary care setting. To improve recognition of persons who might benefit from mental health care, some primary care clinics have implemented the routine use of screening instruments to detect common problems such as depression and alcohol abuse. An easy-to-administer screen for depression in primary care that consists of two verbally asked questions, one regarding depressed mood and the other regarding loss of interest, has been shown to have high diagnostic sensitivity and specificity (Arroll et al. 2003). A study to assess the use of screening for alcoholism in primary care within the large Veterans Affairs health system found that 85% of primary care patients received some form of screening for alcoholism, the predominant screen being the CAGE questions (Barry et al. 2004). Inservice talks to primary care staff about the recognition of psychiatric illness provided by mental health staff, for example at staff meetings, can improve case finding as well. Finally, the mere co-location of mental health staff within primary care, uniformly present and readily available to help on a consistent basis, will naturally encourage primary care providers to inquire about the psychosocial needs of their patients. Primary care providers, on the other hand, may be less likely to ask patients about mental illness or social need if they fear this will open a Pandora's box of problems that they have neither training, time, or referral access to manage.

Once case identification has occurred, the manner in which a primary care doctor or nurse practitioner makes a referral to mental health care will affect the success of that referral. In addition to declining referral because of denial of illness, patients may be influenced by anxiety, previous negative experiences in mental health care, and the effects of stigma regarding mental illness. In this spirit, directly introducing the mental health clinician to the patient as a full member of the primary care team reduces the shame and fear associated with seeing a mental health provider. The referring clinician should be on the lookout for body language or other evidence that the patient is reluctant to accept the referral. The primary care psychiatrist should encourage and, if necessary, coach the referring primary care clinician to explore this reluctance with gentle, open-ended questions regarding the patient's feelings about seeing a mental health provider. When patients decline mental health care outright, the co-located mental health specialists may continue to collaborate with the referring provider to discuss the case and provide behind-the-scenes guidance as needed.

UNIQUE ASPECTS OF THE PRIMARY CARE SETTING

When treating mentally ill homeless people in primary care, incongruence can exist between a primary care clinician's mission—to provide comprehensive, thorough treatment and health maintenance care—and a homeless patient's goal of meeting immediate survival needs. This is illustrated by juxtaposing the elderly, homeless Mr. L's chief complaint, "I need help," with the triage note that indicated he came "without a clear reason." These conflicting goals often result in medical staff perceiving homeless mentally ill patients as noncompliant, uncooperative, or untreatable because they did not take the medications as prescribed or follow up as recommended. The patients in this setting may similarly feel that the provider is not interested in helping them with what they truly need and is focused instead on a seemingly unrelated agenda. For example, a homeless patient with diabetes or hypertension who does not feel sick often will not consider attention to that issue a priority. Furthermore, active substance misuse, psychosis, or depression, all common in homeless patients, will generally impede a patient's attention to health maintenance recommendations. Other mentally ill homeless patients may not adhere to primary care recommendations because they do not understand them; this may be due to insufficient explanation, health illiteracy, disorganization of thinking, or psychotic denial of a health problem. Some homeless consumers may enter a provider–consumer treatment relationship with low trust that stems from paranoia, or simply from prior real or perceived disrespect by clinicians, the health facility in general, or other authority figures (Institute of Medicine 1988). In all of these situations, success in implementing health recommendations requires that the provider first establish trust.

Another challenge in providing good care to a homeless mentally ill person in the primary care setting is that many public primary care clinics have a system of appointments that assumes patients have money for transportation, as well as flexibility in their schedules. However, a homeless person with an unstable housing situation may be temporarily residing very far from a clinic, and travel distance combined with transportation costs may deter attendance. If the person is living in a shelter, he or she may be required to return there in the early evening to wait in line to reenter or, similarly, wait in a soup kitchen line to obtain meals. Furthermore, the rescheduling routines and missed-appointment policies at some primary care clinics can seem punitive, especially if patients must wait significant periods for another appointment or, worse, are administratively discharged from the clinic for multiple missed appointments.

DEVELOPING A TREATMENT PLAN

After Mr. L's admission for a myocardial infarction, he was discharged to the primary care clinic yet was repeatedly rehospitalized for recurrent episodes of congestive heart failure. During these multiple medical hospitalizations, the psychiatry service was repeatedly consulted because he was viewed as noncompliant with care, resulting in unnecessary and frequent hospital admissions. The medical house-staff requested assessment and documentation of Mr. L's competency to refuse medications as an outpatient. They also noted that Mr. L was not taking any psychotropic medication, despite his history of schizophrenia, and requested recommendations for an antipsychotic medication to start.

A discussion with Mr. L by the primary care psychiatrist revealed that Mr. L did not understand why he was repeatedly prescribed multiple medications, including a diuretic. He was required to take some of these medications in the morning, some in the afternoon, and some at night. From Mr. L's point of view, he knew that he urinated excessively and urgently after taking them. His street homelessness offered very limited access to bathrooms, and this made his life very difficult. He explained to the psychiatrist that he spent his evenings sitting in fast food restaurants and each morning used the bathroom and shower at a public facility. After about one o'clock in the afternoon each day, he walked the streets until late evening. The psychiatrist and the inpatient medical house-staff team discussed simplifying Mr. L's medication regimen in a way that, while suboptimal in domiciled patients, reduced excessive daytime urination. However, his primary care physician was hesitant to endorse technically suboptimal care, and Mr. L was discharged on the same regimen.

Mr. L continued a pattern of medication nonadherence and rehospitalization, although with each hospitalization the primary care psychiatrist was involved in treatment planning. Over time, the psychiatrist developed an alliance with him, and eventually Mr. L agreed to visit him between hospitalizations at the clinic. Although Mr. L continued to deny that he had a psychiatric illness, he was appreciative of the support and human contact and stopped by periodically to talk.

A primary care treatment plan in a homeless mentally ill person should focus on goals and objectives that are reasonable when taking into account the person's current social and psychiatric challenges. The steps we discuss in this chapter do require time, frequently a real-world premium commodity for primary care clinicians. For this reason, we underscore the need for ongoing multidisciplinary care, using psychiatry, social work, and often nursing as well, to weave a health care support system around patients with very complex problems.

The plan should be broad and should include input from staff in a variety of disciplines who have expertise in the patient's general medical, psychiatric, and social needs. Trust building, or engagement, is a first step. This occurs through staff's taking a nonjudgmental, helpful approach and understanding the patient's needs as he or she sees them. The priority of achieving stable housing is key, and it is important that all members of the interdisciplinary team maintain awareness of the primacy of this rehabilitation goal.

Continuity of care within the team is highly beneficial in establishing a trusting treatment relationship with consistent primary care and mental health providers. If a patient is hospitalized, the primary care clinician and psychiatrist should be involved in conceptualizing the plan for inpatient care, discharge planning, and follow-up.

Planning for outpatient medical and mental health appointments for a homeless patient must also take into account limitations posed by homelessness. For instance, clinics cannot generally telephone a homeless person to arrange a follow-up or specialty appointment. Rather, all appointments must be offered at the time of a primary appointment. To encourage attendance, car fare should also be provided. This may require a referral to the clinic social worker. Alternatively, a system of open access, which allows some patients the flexibility to come in for care when they are able to, may be more effective.

When planning care for primary medical problems of a mentally ill homeless patient, a provider must take special care to clarify any gaps in understanding of the clinical assessment and recommendations. Any reluctance about the latter should be gently explored in an open, nonjudgmental way. When patients are nonadherent or reluctant to accept provider recommendations, primary care psychiatrists can help primary care clinicians adopt a Stages of Change model to conceptualize a patient's position in terms of readiness to make health-promoting decisions (Prochaska et al. 1992; Zimmerman et al. 2000). This approach, combined with motivational interviewing techniques to gently advance behavioral health change readiness over time, optimizes the chances of producing positive results (Rollnick 1996). A consulting psychiatrist may be asked to evaluate a nonadherent patient's capacity to refuse care, as in the case of Mr. L. Rather than providing a simple statement on capacity, however, it is generally more useful that the psychiatrist redirect the focus of evaluation and intervention toward understanding barriers to adherence and devising strategies for engagement in care.

In more extreme cases, the psychiatric consultant may be called to evaluate the capacity of an acutely medically unstable patient who refuses medical admission through the emergency department—or, once hospitalized, refuses critically important procedures or is leaving the hospital against medical advice. This behavior is more commonly seen in homeless patients whose reasoning is affected by psychotic thinking or craving for alcohol or an illicit substance. In making recommendations, the consulting psychiatrist must weigh 1) the severity and acuity of the medical disorder as determined by the primary medical provider, 2) the expected value of involuntary medical admission in a patient who may continue to refuse medications or evaluative procedures once admitted, and 3) possible exacerbation of the person's fear of the health care system through forced hospitalization or treatment. In some cases, involuntary admission to inpatient psychiatric care is justifiable on the basis of the patient's inability to think through critically important medical decisions owing to a treatable psychiatric condition. One goal in these cases is to restore the patient's capacity to make autonomous decisions.

When patients do agree to take medication of any kind, prescription must take into account the patient's living situation. Whenever possible, the number of medications and dosing frequency should be simplified and tailored to what is very practical. For Mr. L, his diuretic's side effect of producing much urination had a compounded effect of his declining all medications, unsure which one was causing this side effect. If medications are prescribed during an outpatient visit, they should be provided to that patient on that very day, ideally at the time of the visit. Without significant case management support, a homeless patient is less likely to receive medications if he or she must return to the facility for them, make a copayment, or receive them through mail. Obtaining medications for homeless patients without relevant benefits may be especially difficult. Most pharmaceutical programs offer medication assistance programs to provide free medication for those who have no prescription drug coverage and whose income falls below certain levels. Such programs generally require initiation by the prescribing physician, documented evidence of financial hardship, and reapplication for the medication every few months (Chisholm and DiPiro 2002). Whenever homeless patients are prescribed medication, inquiry concerning adherence should be regularly made at follow-up visits and barriers to adherence explored.

Regarding psychiatric treatment in primary care, patients should not be pressured to take psychotropic medications or even to accept a psychiatric referral. Such action can be perceived as judgmental and can damage the therapeutic alliance. In these cases, a primary care provider may "curbside" the on-site mental health provider when important questions arise and can otherwise be encouraged to continue to work on establishing trust with that patient, biding time for later discussion of mental health problems.

ACCESS TO ENTITLEMENTS

The social worker engaging homeless people in a primary care setting should be a mental health specialist. Sometimes this professional is the first mental health clinician to meet with mentally ill homeless clients in this setting. The meeting may occur through referral by the primary care provider for social work services—or for mental health consultation, in a system where a psychiatric social worker triages all new referrals. In a shelter-based primary care clinic, the social worker may also be the very first allied health provider to have contact with the homeless person, often while orienting him or her to the new shelter system. As in the case of a psychiatrist or psychiatric nurse practitioner, collaboration with the primary care staff must be emphasized.

The social worker in primary care has a variety of roles. This professional is often the bridge to psychiatric consultation and therefore serves as a key facilitator and engagement specialist. Once the patient is in treatment, the social worker reinforces adherence to a psychiatric regimen and offers concrete help in doing so, such as filling prescriptions and acting as liaison to the medical staff. As part of a case management role, the social worker focuses on necessary entitlements, especially health insurance, and facilitates continuity of care as clients change shelters or living situations. This phase includes ensuring that health care records accompany the patient with a change of care settings. Supportive counseling is yet another role, addressing adjustment issues, building adaptive skills, discussing vocational goals, and acting as the patient's prime agent in achieving the crucial goal of gaining housing.

Some homeless clients may be reluctant to accept a referral for housing from a social worker. Paranoid patients may avoid group living settings because they are afraid of persecution; other patients fear the loss of freedom that may accompany a supportive living setting; some do not want to contribute the money that may be required for housing. Homeless patients may also fear the changes associated with more independent housing, including greater responsibility, isolation, or the loss of a peer group that they may have had while homeless. The mental health clinician in primary care who gains the trust of a mentally ill homeless client may eventually serve as a bridge connecting the client to housing and social services.

One day, Mr. L presented to the office of the primary care psychiatrist in distress, crying, and stated that he was tired of being on the street and felt desperate to find a place to live. Previously he had declined a social work services referral for housing because of his fears of persecution by other residents in a shared-living setting. However, on this occasion, Mr. L agreed that his psychiatrist could make some phone calls with him and arrange a meeting with a psychiatric social worker who specialized in housing homeless persons. Mr. L subsequently initiated the paperwork to apply for a housing program, and by the time of his next hospitalization for heart failure, he was successfully discharged into a shared-room program.

REFERENCES

Arroll B, Khin N, Kerse N: Screening for depression in primary care with two verbally asked questions: cross sectional study. BMJ 327:1144–1146, 2003

Barry KL, Blow FC, Willenbring ML, et al: Use of alcohol screening and brief interventions in primary care settings: implementation and barriers. Subst Abus 25:27–36, 2004

Chisholm MA, DiPiro JT: Pharmaceutical manufacturer assistance programs. Arch Intern Med 162:780–784, 2002

Institute of Medicine, Committee on Health Care for Homeless People: Homelessness, Health and Human Needs. Washington, DC, National Academy Press, 1988

Prochaska JO, DiClemente CC, Norcross JC: In search of how people change: applications to addictive behaviors. Am Psychol 47:1102–1114, 1992

Rollnick S: Behaviour change in practice: targeting individuals. Int J Obes Relat Metab Disord 20 (suppl 1):S22–S26, 1996

Sullivan MD, Cole SA, Gordon GF, et al: Psychiatric training in medicine residencies: current needs, practices, and satisfaction. Gen Hosp Psychiatry 18:95–101, 1996

Wedding D, Mengel M: Models of integrated care in primary care settings, in Handbook of Primary Care Psychology. Edited by Haas LJ. New York, Oxford University Press, 2004, pp 47–60

Zimmerman GL, Olsen CG, Bosworth MF: A "stages of change" approach to helping patients change behavior. Am Fam Physician 61:1409–1416, 2000

Chapter 11

HOMELESS CHILDREN

Manoj Shah, M.D.
Randie Schacter, D.O.

On initial presentation, Mary was 14 years old and came to the emergency department alone complaining of fever and severe abdominal pain. On assessment, her findings were consistent with pelvic inflammatory disease, and the medical workup revealed gonorrhea as its cause. She was admitted. During her admission, she revealed she had run away from home about a month earlier to escape chaos and violence. Her mother's live-in boyfriend was physically abusing her mother, her two siblings, and Mary as well. During Mary's month of homelessness, a stranger befriended her. He also began to abuse her physically and sexually and became her pimp. She had been alone and frightened, and he threatened to harm her if she disclosed her predicament to anyone. Eventually the symptoms of her pelvic inflammatory disease became so bad that she turned to the emergency room for help.

During her hospitalization, the inpatient evaluation revealed also symptoms of posttraumatic stress disorder and depression. She was transferred to the psychiatry service. Using a multidisciplinary approach, the inpatient team was able to coordinate contact with her mother. At the time, mother and siblings were living in a shelter. The hospital social worker worked with the shelter social worker to access entitlements such as Medicaid and Social Security for Mary. They also arranged for outpatient follow-up for her medical problems and psychiatric disorders.

Mary's case illustrates homelessness among children and youth as a significant issue often occurring within stressed, impoverished families, degrading the fabric of our communities. Studies show that the most impoverished children in our society are often homeless (Rossi 1989). They also note that poor and/or homeless children are more likely to have emotional and behavioral problems if their mother is emotionally distressed (Rossi 1989). As medical professionals, we should be familiar with the magnitude of this problem and the steps needed to aid children and families most efficiently. It is estimated that 1.35 million children experience homelessness in a given year in the United States (Urban Institute 2000), most of whom are of preschool and elementary school ages (U.S. Department of Education 2003).

CHARACTERISTICS OF HOMELESS CHILDREN AND YOUTH

When considering homeless children, it is easier to address their issues with regard to risk factors, supports, and needs by separating them into two categories: those who are homeless with their parents and those who are homeless on their own. It is more common for young children to be homeless with a parent than alone. For example, in a study by Rog and colleagues (1995), the authors noted that in nine major American cities that they reviewed, the typical homeless family consisted of a single mother in her early 30s with two children under the age of five (see Chapter 4, Homeless Families in Shelters).

Homelessness has a particularly detrimental effect on children when they are alone. They have unstable lives and often lack medical care. The insufficient living conditions tend to increase these young people's vulnerability to chronic illnesses like ear or respiratory infections, gastrointestinal disorders, and sexually transmitted diseases, including HIV/AIDS. In fact, homeless children are twice as likely to develop a medical ailment as other children (Better Homes Fund 1999). They have also been found to experience more mental health problems such as anxiety, depression, and withdrawal (Better Homes Fund 1999). A study by Redlener and Johnson (1999) in New York City revealed that only 39% of children without housing have received their proper immunizations, compared with 77% of all New York 2-year-olds. This finding affects not only these children but also those who interact with them. The 38% asthma rate of children in this study of sheltered children was four times that of all New York City children. In the same study, the authors also noted that the rate of ear infection was 50% greater than the national average. When taking into consideration the lack of medical care that these children receive, the risk of poorly managed ear infections has the potential to result in deafness and learning problems that can snowball into increased school dropout rates and criminal behavior. This affects all of society, not just these young people.

Teenagers are at greater risk for homelessness than are younger children because of running away or being abandoned (Hammer et al. 2002). Causes of homelessness in this population are often complex. They include strained family relationships that result in communication problems; abuse and neglect; parental substance abuse; and mental health problems. "Throwaways" or runaways can emerge from such situations. Hammer and colleagues (2002) noted that in a 1999 study 1,680,000 youths had a runaway or throw-away episode. In only 37% of these cases did the parents attempt to find the child, and only 21% of these adolescents were reported to the authorities as missing. Gay and lesbian youth and pregnant teens are a vulnerable population, leaving their families prematurely and becoming homeless. Economic crises and family disbanding are other causes of youth homelessness. Additional causes include instability of residential placements like foster care, including the problem of "aging out" of foster care systems and residential schools and juvenile detention (Camino and Epley 1998; Robertson 1991). Moreover, this population has unique complications regarding legal status as minors in terms of accessing services, employment, housing, and other resources (Robertson 1991). To survive on the streets, homeless children often resort to prostitution, drug trafficking, and other forms of criminal behavior (Janus et al. 1987). They are also likely to be victims of physical and sexual exploitation, yielding a higher risk of posttraumatic stress disorder (PTSD) and other comorbid mental health problems (Cauce et al. 2000; Davidson et al. 1991; Janus et al. 1987; Kipke et al. 1997).

CLINICAL ENGAGEMENT

> Mary showed symptoms of PTSD, such as nightmares, hypervigilance, and avoidance. These were accompanied by depressed mood, with hopelessness, suicidal ideation, and severe insomnia. She had been vulnerable to street predators in addition to being sexually and physically abused by her pimp.

In medical settings, a homeless child or adolescent is most likely to be encountered by a mental health professional in an emergency department or as part of a consultation on a pediatric medical unit. Often the child has limited access to medical care and has come in on an emergency basis because a physical illness has worsened. Once the child is in the medical system, it is vitally important for the psychiatrist or other mental health professional to engage these children and, if possible, their families. This requires a team approach, usually consisting of a pediatrician, psychiatrist, psychologist, and social worker.

When addressing homeless children, the clinician must take a supportive, nonpunitive, and nonjudgmental stance. It is important to explain that the goal is to help set up a support structure that will improve the child's current living situation and medical issues. Multiple separate visits over several days are likely to improve rapport and to yield more information with regard to the child's living situation, history, and needs.

If, despite being on the streets, the child is accompanied by the parent in the medical setting, the child must have the opportunity to speak to the health care provider alone at some point near the beginning of the evaluation. This serves to enhance the child's engagement and affords an opportunity to share information the child may not feel comfortable imparting when caretakers are present. However, this situation must be approached with great sensitivity. The child may actually be reluctant to speak without the guardian present. Children in this situation may be frightened that the parent will abandon them or get angry at them for disclosing anything, or even fear that disclosure may get the parent in trouble. The initial solo contact is therefore usually short and acts as an icebreaker, setting the stage for subsequent interaction and information gathering. Follow-up should occur promptly, either later the same day or during the very next day, encouraging the child's sense of continuity and support.

It is common for homeless children to be untrusting and to avoid eye contact. Consider how they must feel after being subjected to so many daily hardships and inconsistencies. Empathic validation of the child's feelings, and the guardian's too, often leads to disclosure of current and past experiences that are relevant to understanding the current clinical situation. It is also important to normalize the experience for children, with ample explanation that the clinician has worked with other homeless children, has been able to help them, can understand their concerns and fears, and has confidence that these concerns and fears can be constructively addressed.

These principles apply to adolescents, too. When dealing with homeless adolescents, one is even more likely to encounter a lack of trust in authority or elders. This is developmentally normative, but "street kids" frequently have no sense of security, protection, or hope. They often are used to being chastised by authorities: yelled at for lying in doorways or on benches in public areas. Exacerbating their alienation is the fact that they are most likely victims of abuse or abandonment by their guardians (Youth Advocacy Program International 2005) and then are further victimized on the street, as we have seen in Mary's situation. Clarity and understanding will take the clinician farther than paternalism (Youth Advocacy Program International 2005). It is important to maintain good eye contact with adolescents and to be honest about what will happen during the course of their care, seeking to maximize the transparency of intentions.

THE PSYCHIATRIC INTERVIEW: DIFFERENTIAL DIAGNOSIS

When discussing sensitive areas of the interview such as abuse and neglect, using open-ended questions will elicit the most information and, importantly, will prevent leading the child to say what he or she thinks the interviewer wants to hear. For younger children, asking questions like "Has anyone ever hit you or hurt you? Who? Where and how?" and then offering an empathic comment is helpful. It allows them to feel comfortable with their disclosure, increasing the likelihood that they will talk more. With regard to sexual abuse in the younger groups, specifically ask if anyone has touched their "private parts" or touched them "down there" (while pointing to where the interviewer is referring). If the answer is affirmative, then the interviewer must not ask leading questions and must resist comments that fill in informational blanks but instead should ask the child to describe the experience and who did it to him or her. The power of suggestion is strong in the younger ages, especially.

With older youth, being matter-of-fact in questioning, yet empathic with regard to their answers, is also helpful. It is important to clarify terms and to ensure that questions are understood, avoiding a situation in which the patient "yes's" the interviewer to avoid admitting to not understanding. When asking about sexual activity, it is important to ask about the patient's definition of "having sex." For example, some youth do not identify oral sex with sexual activity. A history of current sexual behavior is important because many homeless youths engage in sex at higher rates and at younger ages ("Early Family Abuse" 2001) than domiciled young people.

The psychiatric interview of homeless children and adolescents includes all phases of a conventional psychiatric evaluation, with special attention to factors specific to this population. Table 11–1 summarizes the points covered in the psychiatric interview.

It is our experience that a successful and comprehensive evaluation will emerge with use of the techniques we have described. While using these techniques, the psychiatrist maintains heightened sensitivity to the presence of anxiety, depression, and withdrawal, syndromes common to this population (Bassuk et al. 2005). As noted, the history must cover present and past neglect and physical and sexual abuse. A thorough psychosocial assessment is essential, focusing on the current living situation and how homelessness occurred, with special consideration of how such issues affect decisions on disposition. For example, a runaway teenager whose home is unsafe will need a different plan than a child homeless with his or her parent. School enrollment and attendance history should be explored in the light of poor attendance and lack of enrollment that may be directly related to the child's homelessness (National Coalition for the Homeless 2005). When addressing past psychiatric history, it is important to consider whether the prohibitive cost of medication is a factor in lack of adherence and how best to overcome this problem, either through Medicaid application or drug company–sponsored patient assistance programs. Substance and alcohol misuse is important as well. Studies have found that up to 90% of homeless children use psychoactive substances, which include medicines, alcohol, cigarettes, heroin, cannabis, and industrial products like shoe glue and paint (Youth Advocacy Program International 2005). When children are living with their families, assessing parental risk of substance abuse and mental illness is also important. Mental illness and sub-

TABLE 11–1.   Interview checklist

Psychosocial evaluation
   Previous household constellation
   History of abuse
      Physical
      Sexual
      Neglect
   School history
      Learning disorder
      Mental retardation
      Attendance history
   Substance use (including cigarettes)
      Parents
      Sibling
      Patient
   Sexual history
      Pregnancy/abortion
      Sexually transmitted diseases
   Legal issues
   Family psychiatric history

Mental status
   Anxiety
   Depression
   Posttraumatic stress disorder
   Avoidance
   Paranoia
   Suicidal attempts and current status

Medical evaluation
   Hygiene
   Nutritional status
   Infection (ear)
   Hearing
   Vision
   Dental
   Asthma
   Vaccines
   Laboratory
      Complete blood count
      Comprehensive metabolic panel
      Pregnancy
      Toxicology
      Sexually transmitted diseases
      HIV/AIDS
      Drug screen

stance abuse have heritable factors that put children at risk, and prevention and psychoeducation can be helpful. Providing referrals for parents can assist in stabilizing the family success and reducing homelessness. Prevention also may require the involvement of child protective agencies for neglect issues related to substance abuse and mental illness (Rosenheck et al. 1999).

Homeless children are more likely to have developmental delays (Rosenheck et al. 1999). Addressing developmental milestones, including speech and cognition, is therefore particularly important in formulating appropriate educational, rehabilitative, and clinical interventions. Related hygiene and nutritional status are part of this assessment.

MEDICAL EVALUATION

The necessary medical workup explores the potential physiologic sequelae related to the risk factors associated with homelessness. A medical exam includes attention to nutrition and hygiene. In addition, factors that may be contributing to or complicating any nonpsychiatric illness should be investigated via laboratory tests. A complete blood count, comprehensive chemistry screen, pregnancy test, toxicology, and screens for sexually transmitted diseases, including HIV, are important initial tests. Immunization history, vision, hearing, and dental examination must also be covered. Once the exam is completed, a treatment plan to address the medical findings will be needed. Ideally, a review of findings and consensus on discharge planning occur in a team meeting involving the psychiatrist, social worker, and medical team. When acting as a consultant, the psychiatric clinician speaks about findings and recommendations directly with the requesting physician, and any ideas for management, during the hospitalization and afterward, should be included in the written consultation. If the child is a psychiatric inpatient, it is important for the psychiatrist to confirm with pediatric consultants what aspects of their evaluations must be completed in the hospital and which are planned on an outpatient basis. Social work can play a critical role in avoiding a poorly coordinated follow-up. For example, for children who live in shelters, the hospital social worker confirms that the shelter's caseworker is aware of the child's medical issues and also communicates the findings to the doctor who provides services to the shelter's residents.

SOCIAL SERVICES EVALUATION

Social work services are indispensable. This discipline further addresses parental involvement, the family's social and financial resources, abuse/neglect histories, and academic issues. The social worker also coordinates with court-appointed legal guardians assigned through the community's child protective services agency. The role of the social worker is to gather information on all of these issues and then work with the team to design comprehensive and truly viable treatment and disposition plans. The social worker also has a special relationship with the psychiatrist (with their specific role depending on their respective skill sets) in planning and carrying out family systems interventions, including psychoeducation and family therapy, with the patient and caretakers.

DEVELOPING A TREATMENT PLAN

A comprehensive treatment plan incorporates psychiatric recommendations with those of other involved disciplines. The psychiatric practitioner as a team member is uniquely poised to help integrate the emerging treatment and service plan within a biopsychosocial framework.

Treatment plans are by definition flexible. As current and historical details emerge, plans may change. For a child in need of emergent treatment when a parent is not available, for example, the treatment team takes appropriate initiative. With regard to psychiatric issues, it is noteworthy that a child is allowed an evaluation without parental consent if the child has shown any behavior that is life-threatening and needs acute management for safety reasons. As clinical stability is achieved, seeking out parental consent is necessary whenever possible. Otherwise, clinicians must have available to them an institutional ethics and legal apparatus to determine whether the minor can consent to treatment in the absence of the parent or whether local governmental child protective services must be involved, acting as legal guardian. Predicting potential complications in advance facilitates the treatment process. In Mary's case, being able to contact her mother allowed the hospital to obtain consent to continue treatment and arrange appropriate transition in treatment and other services.

ACCESSING ENTITLEMENTS
Medicaid and Social Security

We have already mentioned that ongoing psychiatric and medical interventions cannot proceed without a viable context in which they may be delivered. The patient and family (if involved) must obviously have access to basic needs, like food and clothing. The team's dispositional or transition plan must account for this and may include application for Supplemental Security Income (SSI) or Medicaid, as appropriate, with resources for clothing and nutrition and Social Security benefits. Disability benefits and medical coverage are helpful in accessing rehabilitation services. (Please note that a child does not qualify for SSDI benefits.) As for qualification, a child under age 18 can qualify for SSI (not SSDI) benefits if he or she meets Social Security's definition of disability for children in that the child's mental or physical condition results in "marked and severe functional limitations" and must have lasted or is expected to last for at least 12 months (examples: total blindness or deafness, cerebral palsy, severe mental retardation) and the child's income and resources have to fall within the eligibility limits (U.S. Social Security Administration 2005). Medical coverage is provided through the state in which the child resides, either via Medicaid or through the State Children's Health Insurance Program if the child's or the parents' income is too high for Medicaid eligibility (U.S. Department of Health and Human Services 2005). Medical coverage from either of these sources requires a separate application than those filed for other benefits (U.S. Social Security Administration 2005).

Housing

Housing is another basic resource. For homeless youth, housing issues are often complicated, since many shelters require a guardian. Housing for youth potentially can be achieved through family reunification or placement in foster or group homes. However, this is often a turbulent transition for street youth as they move from no structure at all to necessarily structured settings. For many older youths with serious emotional disorders, including those "aging out" of the child welfare system, "foyer" independent living programs, pioneered with success in Europe, offer the type of flexible engagement that enables a transition to stability and social reintegration (YMCA England 2005). These housing programs offer housing and individualized and psychosocial support during a uniquely transitional life phase (Good Shepherd Services 2005).

School

School enrollment should be facilitated. The psychiatric evaluation, recommendations, and plan should be forwarded to the school system, along with a special education evaluation request from the child's guardian. This will assist in providing the child with necessary support services in school and increase the likelihood that the child will succeed despite the turbulence that occurred prior to mental health intervention.

Mental Health and Chemical Dependency Treatment

Concerning mental health follow-up, issues of abuse, abandonment, and self-esteem are often key clinical factors to be addressed in selecting appropriate services. Psychoeducation is also critical. Explaining to the patient and the guardian the evaluation and treatment recommendations will increase adherence to recommended outpatient psychiatric care, appropriate medication management and psychotherapy, and family supports. It is important to review the detailed recommendations slowly and carefully with the patient and guardian, assessing understanding of the plan, while emphasizing a collaborative approach. As discussed earlier, a family history of substance abuse is common and heritable in this population. Assisting affected family members in obtaining treatment will likely improve outcome. Psychoeducation (without a lecturing attitude) regarding the nature and consequences of abuse may be helpful.

Portable Medical Records

Finally, among the many stressors facing this group, movement from place to place with tenuous community ties often leads to poorly directed follow-up and a fragmented case history. In an effort to improve treatment, the social worker should create a portable medical record. Gathering prior evaluations (e.g., psychiatric, psychological, medical, immunization, vision, hearing, dental, special education) and past medical studies into one packet is a very important service. This medical record is given to the patient or the guardian and sent to the pediatrician or other primary service provider to whom the patient will be referred. In addition to preventing useless repetition of lab tests and studies, it also communicates a goal-oriented approach to rehabilitation to the patient and to the treatment team to which the patient's services are transferred.

CONCLUSION

The assessment and successful management of a homeless child requires the clinician to be sensitive, patient, and knowledgeable about the child's special needs. Engaging a homeless child without parents differs from working with a child in a homeless family in that the clinician has to interact with multiple agencies and learn to work in a multidisciplinary team. The psychiatrist's role by default becomes that of a coordinator or a team leader. A close working relationship between the psychiatrist and the social worker is particularly important to help negotiate the multiple agencies and to develop and implement a comprehensive treatment plan. These children are extremely needy, they have been traumatized, and they need time, patience, and a warm, caring, gentle approach to develop trust. They also need treatment plan follow-through to achieve a successful outcome. Each child must be handled as an individual with unique needs, and the treatment plan must reflect this. The

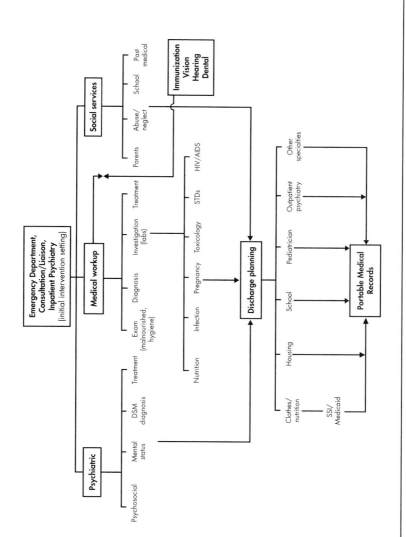

FIGURE 11–1. Flowchart of evaluation and plan consideration in homeless children.

checklist and flowchart in this chapter serve as guides (see Table 11–1 and Figure 11–1), but the customized treatment and management plan requires creative development. The inpatient contact is only the first step in a long journey. For the plan to succeed, an adequate follow-up is essential. The theologian Dietrich Bonhoeffer said, "the test of the morality of a society is what it does for its children." In the case of homeless children, any systemic failure to help the child complete the journey is catastrophic for the child, for his or her family, and for society.

REFERENCES

Bassuk EL, Friedman SM, et al: Facts on Trauma and Homeless Children. Homelessness and Extreme Poverty Working Group, National Child Traumatic Stress Network, 2005. Available at: http://www.nctsnet.org/nctsn_assets/pdfs/promising_practices/Facts_on_Trauma_and_Homeless_Children.pdf. Accessed December 22, 2005.

Better Homes Fund: Homeless Children: America's New Outcasts, Newton Centre, MA, Better Homes Fund, 1999

Camino LA, Epley KA: Having a place to call home. Paper presented at the National Network for Youth and W. K. Kellogg Foundation Conference, Washington, DC, April 7–9, 1998

Cauce AM, Paradise M, Ginzler JA, et al: The characteristics and mental health of homeless adolescents: age and gender differences. J Emotion Behav Disord 8:230–239, 2000

Davidson JR, Hughes D, Blazer DG, et al: Post-traumatic stress disorder in the community: an epidemiological study. Psychol Med 21:713–721, 1991

Early family abuse indirectly increased STD risk among homeless and runaway youth. RAP Time, Vol 5, April 2001. Available at: http://www.indiana.edu/~aids/V5no4p65.pdf. Accessed October 15, 2005.

Good Shepherd Services: The Foyer nine months later. Available at: http://www.goodshepherds.org/sub-news_events/ne-news_article.php?art=461. Accessed December 17, 2005.

Hammer H, Finkelhor D, Sedlak A: Runaway/thrownaway children: national estimates and characteristics. National incidence studies of missing, abducted, runaway, and thrownaway children, 2002. Available at: http://www.ncjrs.org/html/ojjdp/nismart/04/. Accessed October 15, 2005.

Janus MD, Burgess AW, McCormack A: Histories of sexual abuse in adolescent male runaways. Adolescence 22:405–417, 1987

Kipke MD, Simon TR, Montgomery SB, et al: Homeless youth and their exposure to and involvement in violence while living on the streets. J Adolesc Health 20:360–367, 1997

National Coalition for the Homeless: Fact Sheet: Bringing America Home. Available at: http://www.bringingamericahome.org/education.html. Accessed October 15, 2005.

Redlener I, Johnson D: Still in crisis: the health status of New York's homeless children. New York, Children's Health Fund, 1999

Robertson M: Homeless youths: an overview of recent literature, in Homeless Children and Youth: A New American Dilemma. Edited by Kryder-Coe J, Salmon L, Molnar J. New Brunswick, NJ, and London, Transaction, 1991, pp 33–68

Rog DJ, McCombs-Thornton KL, Gilbert-Mongelli AM, et al: Implementation of the Homeless Families Program, 2: characteristics, strengths, and needs of participant families. Am J Orthopsychiatry 65:514–528, 1995

Rosenheck R, Bassuk E, Salomon A: Special populations of homeless Americans, in Practical Lessons: The 1998 National Symposium on Homelessness Research. Edited by Fosburg LB, Dennis DL. Washington, DC, U.S. Department of Housing and Urban Development and U.S. Department of Health and Human Services, 1999. Available at: http://aspe.hhs.gov/progsys/homeless/symposium/2-Spclpop.htm.

Rossi PH: Down and Out in America: The Origins of Homelessness. Chicago, IL, University of Chicago Press, 1989

Urban Institute: A New Look at Homelessness in America. February 1, 2000. Washington, DC, Urban Institute, 2000

U.S. Census Bureau: 2003. Available at: http://www.census.gov. Accessed October 15, 2005.

U.S. Department of Education: Report to the President and Congress on the implementation of the Education for Homeless Children and Youth Program under the McKinney-Vento Homeless Assistance Act, September 4, 2004. Available at: http://www.ed.gov/programs/homeless/rpt2006.doc.

U.S. Department of Health and Human Services: Insure Kids Now! Available at: http://www.insurekidsnow.gov. Accessed December 22, 2005.

U.S. Social Security Administration: Benefits for Children With Disabilities. Available at: http://www.ssa.gov/pubs/10026.html. Accessed December 22, 2005.

YMCA England: Moving Out, Moving On: From Foyer Accommodation to Independent Living. Available at: http://www.ymca.org.uk/bfora/systems/xmlviewer/default.asp?arg=DS_YMCA_ABOUTART_38/_page.xsl/34. Accessed December 17, 2005.

Youth Advocacy Program International: Street children and homelessness: the effects of street and homeless life. Available at: http://www.yapi.org/street. Accessed December 22, 2005.

Chapter 12

JAILS AND PRISONS

Erik Roskes, M.D.
Fred Osher, M.D.

Mr. C is a 50-year-old man referred to community mental health services by his probation officer about 3 months prior to his release from a distant federal prison. Mr. C had served about 10 years of his 15-year sentence for bank robbery. Previously, at age 18, while homeless, he was convicted in state court of manslaughter for killing his grandmother while intoxicated and apparently psychotic. Mr. C served 10 years in state prison for the manslaughter charge; during this incarceration, his psychosis and alcohol abuse were not addressed. Released without discharge planning, recommendations to pursue treatment, or housing, he was homeless after release. The bank robbery occurred just 6 months after his release from state prison.

During his second long-term incarceration, Mr. C was diagnosed with schizophrenia and alcohol dependence. There was an effort to link Mr. C to community services prior to his release date, but his probation officer was unable to secure housing before release. However, several crisis placements were arranged (including a VA hospitalization, placement in a crisis respite setting, and the use of a Prisoners' Aid shelter). Mr. C was eventually accepted into a residential and psychosocial rehabilitation program. In collaboration with his psychiatrist and therapist, he was successful in completing his term of probation, and he remains in active treatment within the community mental health system.

OVERVIEW OF CORRECTIONAL SETTINGS

Individuals who are homeless and who have serious mental illnesses are at high risk of incarceration. There are over 11 million "bookings" of individuals into U.S. jails each year (Stephen 2001). The overrepresentation of persons with mental illnesses and substance use disorders in criminal justice settings is well documented (Teplin 1994; Teplin et al. 1996), and almost three-quarters of justice-involved persons with mental illnesses have co-occurring

131

substance use disorders (National GAINS Center 2001; New Freedom Commission 2004). In the year prior to their arrest, 18.6% of inmates with mental illness in federal prison were homeless, compared with 3.2% of other inmates. In local jails, 30.3% of inmates with mental illness were homeless in the year prior to arrest compared with 17.3% of other inmates (Stephen 2001). Michaels et al. (1992) found that 20% of arrested individuals in New York City reported being homeless the night before the arrest. Of those reporting homelessness, 50% had evidence of mental illness, compared with only 25% of those reporting that they had never been homeless.

Reasons for these high rates of homelessness and mental illness among incarcerated populations include society's limited tolerance for the "nuisance" behavior of individuals who are homeless; the difficulty homeless individuals have in accessing quality mental health care and the resultant misbehavior based in their untreated mental illnesses; their high prevalence of co-occurring substance use; and police concern about leaving homeless mentally ill persons on the street (Osher and Han 2002).

On arrest, most often for minor offenses, individuals who cannot or do not make bail are housed in locally operated jails. Jails are designed as short-term detention facilities for individuals who have not yet been tried (and are therefore legally innocent) and also for convicted individuals sentenced to short periods of incarceration, generally less than a year. Individuals found guilty and sentenced to longer terms of incarceration serve those terms in state-run prisons. Unlike jails, which are notable for having very rapid turnover, prisons house only those who have been judged and sentenced, and they tend to have stable populations.

Jails and prisons are obligated to provide general and mental health care (Cohen 1998, 2003; New Freedom Commission 2004) in addition to meeting detainees' other needs. In fact, incarcerated individuals are the only United States citizens with constitutionally protected access to health care. The U.S. Supreme Court, in *Estelle v. Gamble* [429 U.S. 97 (1976)] found that deliberate indifference to prisoners with "serious medical needs" constitutes a violation of the 8th Amendment to the U.S. Constitution. In *Estelle v. Ruiz* [503 F. Supp. 1265 (S.D Tex. 1980)] and subsequent cases, "serious medical needs" were extended by the Fifth Circuit to include mental illness. The Court listed six required components of a minimally acceptable mental health program in a prison:

1. Systematic screening
2. Treatment that is more than segregation and close supervision
3. Treatment that includes the participation of trained mental health professionals who are available in sufficient numbers
4. Accurate, complete, and confidential medical records

5. Prescription of medications in safe manner and with adequate supervision and reevaluation
6. Systematic programming for identification, treatment, and supervision of inmates with suicidal tendencies

The American Association of Community Psychiatrists (AACP; 2001), the American Psychiatric Association (2000), the National Commission on Correctional Health Care (1996, 1997) and the National Institute of Correction (Hills et al. 2004) have all recommended that all jails provide, at minimum, 1) mental health screening, referral, and evaluation; 2) crisis intervention and short-term treatment (most often medication); and 3) discharge and prerelease planning. Of note is that all of these standards include recommendations to ensure connections to adequate housing, in addition to linkage to needed treatment services.

Jails and prisons are far from the optimal venue for the receipt of mental health care. They are chaotic and not well organized for the delivery of high-quality mental health care. Security is the paramount concern. Privacy is difficult and often impossible to find. Mental health staff serves a dual role that includes patient care while also serving the institution's administration. Often, there are strict limits on the number of clinical staff available as well as on the spectrum of available treatments. Nonetheless, the presence of large numbers of homeless persons with mental illnesses in jail presents an opportunity for identification, treatment, and discharge planning that might reduce the far too frequent return to incarceration. In many parts of the country, jails have become psychiatric crisis centers of last resort. Many homeless people and uninsured people with mental illness receive mental health services only in jail because they have been unable to access mental health services in the community. This lack of connection to community mental health services may lead some individuals to cycle through jails dozens or even hundreds of times. Identifying and gaining access to housing is paramount to interrupting this revolving-door cycle.

ROLE OF JAILS AND PRISONS IN THE MANAGEMENT OF MENTAL ILLNESS AMONG HOMELESS PERSONS

Although persons with mental illness are overrepresented within jail populations, many of those individuals had not had contact with mental health providers prior to incarceration. Jails represent a public health outpost where screening, identification, and linkage to community providers are possible, albeit infrequently achieved.

Differential Diagnosis

In the case of Mr. C, for example, the initial failure of the state prison to recognize his co-occurring schizophrenia and alcohol abuse, and the resulting failure to provide appropriate treatment and aftercare planning, undoubtedly led to his committing his second crime. Conversely, as his second incarceration came to a close, the staff expended significant efforts to link him with appropriate community providers, with a vastly better outcome. The institutional intake process presents an opportunity to screen for mental illness along with other problems. Although many jails have a screening mechanism, it most often focuses on suicide assessment and prevention, with an emphasis on reducing the liability of the jailer and the jurisdiction. Screening may consist of as little as one or two questions regarding previous treatment, or it may include a detailed, structured mental status examination. One result of this variability in screening policies is that the many inmates with mental health needs are missed when screened by jail staff (Steadman et al. 2005). Larger jails, in our experience, are more likely to implement their own more comprehensive screening and assessment programs, whereas small jails often rely on local mental health programs or emergency services to provide this service. For example, in New York City any inmate or detainee who is believed by the medical screener or by correctional staff to have mental health needs must be assessed by a mental health provider (generally a social worker or psychiatrist) within 72 hours of the referral. If an acute need is recognized, this assessment will often take place immediately or on the same day. Identification of a homeless person's need for mental health treatment is a critical first step toward community reintegration. Figure 12–1 demonstrates the flow from entry into the jail or prison through the assessment process to transition planning. The figure also outlines the many needs facing inmates and detainees upon release.

Diagnosis can be complex in the correctional setting because inmates often do not trust the providers, instead seeing them as a part of "the system." A high level of clinical skill is required to make accurate diagnoses of substance use and other psychiatric disorders and medical problems. Inmates frequently seek clinical intervention because they have difficulty sleeping in the correctional setting. Sorting out those who are truly symptomatic from those who report symptoms in order to receive sedating medications can be very difficult. Although this phenomenon is not unique to the jail or prison, it poses unique problems within the correctional venue because nearly all psychotropic medications have "street value" within these settings. Given the need to maintain tight security in the correctional institution, it is imperative to have a high degree of both sensitivity and specificity in the diagnostic process: clinicians should strive not to miss those inmates who are mentally ill, and they should also endeavor to rule out mental illness where it does not exist.

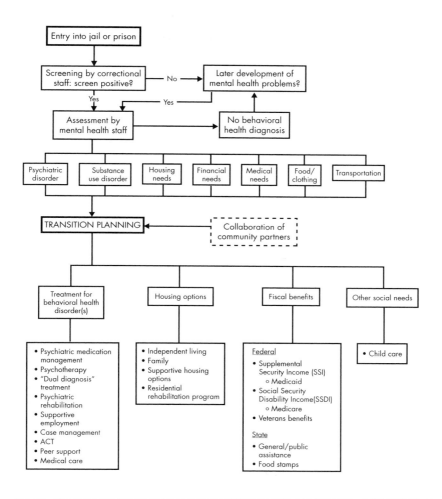

FIGURE 12–1. Flowchart: treatment planning for previously home-less detainees with a mental illness and/or chemical misuse disorders.

Engagement in the Treatment Process

It can also be difficult to identify homeless individuals in this setting, again in part because of inmates' distrust of the staff. The housing status of inmates may vary over the course of an incarceration: inmates who enter the jail believing they can return home may find that they are no longer welcome there, owing at times to the behavior that led to the incarceration. Conversely, inmates believing they are homeless on entry may learn later that a family member is willing to have them return home. Finally, inmates may simply be ashamed to report that they are homeless, or they may falsely report that they are homeless if they believe that by doing so they can get access to new resources.

Nowhere is transition planning more valuable and essential than in jails. Inadequate transition planning puts inmates who entered the jail in a state of crisis back on the streets in the middle of the same crisis. The outcomes of inadequate transition planning include compromised public safety, an increased incidence of psychiatric symptoms, hospitalization, relapse to substance abuse, suicide, ongoing homelessness, and rearrest (Draine and Solomon 1994).

The nature of jails is that there is a relatively short length of stay (weeks to months) with fairly rapid turnover. Short episodes of incarceration in jails (often less then 72 hours) and the often unpredictable nature of jail releases can make discharge or transition planning from jails particularly challenging (AACP 2001, Griffin 1990). A further complication is the uncertain length of any given inmate's incarceration. Pretrial detainees may be bailed out or released from court with little or no notice to clinical providers, making the provision of comprehensive discharge planning very difficult. In unusual cases, an inmate may be civilly committed on release, allowing for more comprehensive treatment and ultimately for discharge planning. However, the majority will be released from jail or court directly into the community. A minority of jail inmates who are serving short sentences may have more predictable release dates; for these inmates, discharge planning is much more straightforward and similar to discharge planning for prisoners.

Accessing Entitlements

A novel response to the problem of unpredictable release times from jail stems from class action litigation in New York, commonly known as the *Brad H.* case. (The Stipulation of Settlement is available at http://www.urbanjustice .org/litigation/index.html). Pursuant to the settlement of this litigation, a comprehensive model of discharge planning that contemplates unpredictable releases was developed and is being implemented in the New York City Department of Correction. In addition to providing access to medications, prescriptions, follow-up mental health care, and benefits, this settlement attends to the housing needs of inmates who report being homeless or who expect to be homeless on release.

Unlike in a jail, release dates for inmates of a prison can often be predicted months or years in advance. These dates can be used as target dates, and mental health staff can have ample time to begin the process of preparing a transition plan. In addition to the case management tasks required, this time can be used to work with the prisoner to prepare him or her for release

(Roskes et al. 2001). Given the relatively long lengths of incarceration, prisoners often are completely divorced from their preincarceration support network, which may need to be rebuilt from scratch.

Without the stability of a bed to sleep on and a roof over one's head, it is difficult to imagine how anyone, particularly someone with a psychiatric problem, can live successfully in the community. The affordable housing crisis in this country makes access to housing extremely limited for people with multiple disabilities, who have a hard time competing for the few available units. In addition, as a result of the federal "one strike and you're out" policy, a person may not be able to rent a federally subsidized apartment if any member of the family has a criminal record. Local housing authorities may develop policies that bar others from Section 8 or other public housing. In addition, states and localities may develop their own statutes. For example, Kansas law prohibits any offender from residing in a group home if he or she is the subject of an insanity finding and is on conditional release from court, jail, prison, or a state mental institution (Kansas Legislature 1996). In addition to these real barriers, there are perceived barriers based largely on preconceived ideas or stigma regarding individuals with criminal histories. For example, even without federal restrictions, landlords may be unwilling to rent a room or apartment to someone with a criminal record.

Finally, it is imperative when preparing an inmate for release to consider not only the housing needs but also the method of paying for that housing, as well as for all other daily needs such as food, clothing, and medications. For individuals who have mental illness, attention should focus primarily on accessing federal benefits such as Supplemental Security Income, Social Security Disability Insurance, and veterans' benefits. Because these benefits often require a significant amount of time and effort before eligibility can be established and payments can begin, jail and prison staff should explore these benefits prior to release. In many instances, it may be much more expedient to seek state sources of funding such as public assistance, general assistance, or welfare benefits, although rarely will these benefits provide adequate funding to cover the cost of housing.

THE COMMUNITY PROVIDER'S RESPONSE TO THE INCARCERATION AND RELEASE OF THE MENTALLY ILL HOMELESS PERSON

Although much of this chapter has focused on the role of providers in the jail or prison setting in developing an aftercare plan, there is also a role to be played by community providers. At the micro level, community providers must be prepared to set aside their prejudice regarding offender populations.

In our experience, although there are exceptions, the vast majority of mentally ill individuals who are released from jails and prisons are not at all unlike the typical population seen by community mental health providers. In fact, studies have found that almost one-half of the clients seen for the first time at community mental health centers have had contact with the criminal justice system, and nearly one-third of them had been sentenced to jail (Theriot and Segal 2005). In many instances, the offense itself, on investigation, can be found to have a basis in symptoms of the mental illness. It is logical to posit that if these individuals are provided with treatment, rehabilitation, and case management for their mental illnesses, and if they are provided with resources to meet their daily needs, the behavior will not recur and the "offender" will be "rehabilitated" in the criminal justice sense of the word.

Community providers will continue to work with persons with criminal justice histories, and so they must become familiar with the terminology of the criminal justice system. This can be done informally, by developing partner relationships with criminal justice professionals (including police officers, parole and probation staff, or judges), or more formally, by taking part in advanced training such as a forensic psychiatry fellowship program. Relationships with criminal justice professionals provide fertile ground for partnering with them in the management of offenders with mental illness and assisting these offenders in reintegrating successfully into the community (see, e.g., Roskes and Feldman 1999; Roskes et al. 1999).

At a macro level, community providers may advocate effectively at the state and local level for improved services and for changes in laws that prevent ex-offenders' access to public mental health services and housing. Not having a home makes participation in court and treatment programs extremely difficult. Homelessness is both a cause of people entering the criminal justice system and an explanatory factor of "revolving door" recidivism. Housing models for people with mental illnesses have been developed, with great success in attaining housing stability. These models typically couple housing with an appropriate level of community support to create a supportive housing program (see Introduction and Chapter 6). Incarcerated offenders with mental illness should receive priority for community public housing resources. Their stability is both a clinical and a public safety concern.

Advocates can get more information from the following Internet sites:

- Council of State Governments (http://www.consensusproject.org)
- American Psychiatric Association, Corresponding Committee on Jails and Prisons (http://www.psych.org/edu/other_res/lib_archives/archives/200401.pdf)
- American Association of Community Psychiatrists, Committee on the Mentally Ill Behind Bars (http://www.comm.psych.pitt.edu/finds/mibb.html)

Jails and prisons are not appropriate housing for individuals with serious mental illnesses. Although some with mental illnesses commit serious crimes and must be incarcerated, most persons with psychiatric disorders who cycle in and out of our jails are not criminals requiring punishment, but citizens deserving treatment—thus pointing to a systemic failure. As jails and prisons begin a process to identify housing needs for detainees and inmates with mental illness, and as correctional staff partner with community providers to expand housing opportunities, mental health providers, too, should be able to attend to housing for patients soon to be released from jail or prison—addressing this need with as much vigor as they focus on other aspects of the clinical aftercare plan.

REFERENCES

American Association of Community Psychiatrists: AACP Continuity of Care Guidelines: Best Practices for Managing Transitions Between Levels of Care. 2001. Available at: http://www.comm.psych.pitt.edu/finds/COG.doc .

American Psychiatric Association: Psychiatric Services in Jails and Prisons: A Task Force Report of the American Psychiatric Association, 2nd Edition. Washington, DC, American Psychiatric Association, 2000

Cohen F: The Mentally Disordered Inmate and the Law. Kingston, NJ, Civic Research Institute, 1998

Cohen F: The Mentally Disordered Inmate and the Law: 2003 Cumulative Supplement. Kingston, NJ, Civic Research Institute, 2003.

Draine J, Solomon P: Jail recidivism and the intensity of case management services among homeless persons with mental illness leaving jail. J Psychiatry Law 22:245–260, 1994

Griffin PA: The backdoor of the jail: linking mentally ill offenders to community mental health services, in Jail Diversion for the Mentally Ill: Breaking Through the Barriers. Effectively Addressing the Mental Health Needs of Jail Detainees. Edited by Steadman HJ. Boulder, CO, National Institute of Corrections, 1990, pp 91–107. Available at: http://www.nicic.org/pubs/1990/008754.pdf.

Hills H, Siegfreid C, Ickowitz A: Effective Prison Mental Health Treatment: Guidelines to Expand and Improve Treatment. Available at: http://www.nicic.org. Washington, DC, National Institute of Corrections, May 2004.

Kansas Legislature: KSA 12–736 Article 7 §(c)(2), 1996. Available at: http://www.kslegislature.org/legsrv-statutes/getStatute.do. Accessed April 7, 2005.

Michaels D, Zoloth SR, Alcabes P, et al: Homelessness and indicators of mental illness among inmates in New York City's correctional system. Hosp Community Psychiatry 43:150–155, 1992

National Commission on Correctional Health Care: Standards for Correctional Health Care for Jails, 1996. Available at: http://www.ncchc.org.

National Commission on Correctional Health Care: Standards for Correctional Health Care for Prisons, 1997. Available at: http://www.ncchc.org.

National GAINS Center for People with Co-occurring Disorders in the Justice System: The Prevalence of Co-occurring Mental Illness and Substance Use Disorders in Jails. Fact Sheet Series. Demar, NY, National GAINS Center, 2001

New Freedom Commission on Mental Health, Subcommittee on Criminal Justice: Background Paper (DHHS Publ No SMA-04-3880). Rockville, MD, 2004

Osher F, Han YL: Jails as Housing for Persons with Serious Mental Illnesses. American Jails 16(1): 36–40, 2002

Roskes E, Feldman R: A collaborative community-based treatment program for offenders with mental illness. Psychiatr Serv 50:1614–1619, 1999

Roskes E, Feldman R, Arrington S, et al: A model program for the treatment of mentally ill offenders in the community. Community Ment Health J 35:461–472, 1999

Roskes E, Craig R, Strangman A: A prerelease program for mentally ill inmates. Psychiatr Serv 52:108, 2001

Steadman HJ, Scott JE, Osher F, et al: Validation of the Brief Jail Mental Health Screen. Psychiatr Serv 56:816–822, 2005

Stephen JJ: Census of Jails, 1999. NCJ 18663. Washington, DC, U.S. Department of Justice Programs, Bureau of Justice Statistics, 2001

Teplin LA: Psychiatric and substance use disorders among male urban jail detainees. Am J Public Health 84:290–293, 1994

Teplin LA, Abram KM, McClelland GM: Prevalence of psychiatric disorders among incarcerated women, I: pretrial jail detainees. Arch Gen Psychiatry 53:505–512 [erratum: 53(8):664], 1996

Theriot MT, Segal SP: Involvement with the criminal justice system among new clients at outpatient mental health agencies. Psychiatr Serv 56:179–185, 2005

Chapter 13

HOMELESS VETERANS

Florence Coleman, M.D.
Julie P. Gentile, M.D.
Ann Morrison, M.D.

Ron is a 55-year-old African American man with bipolar disorder and a history of cocaine dependence. This year, for the first time in 10 years, he is celebrating his birthday with his family.

Ron was able to reach the goal of stable housing and personal relationships after referral to the Intensive Psychiatric Community Care (IPCC) program, which is a U.S. Department of Veterans Affairs (VA) version of Assertive Community Treatment (ACT). He was referred after struggling for 20 years with severe mental illness and addiction. He had experienced more than 10 hospitalizations, 3 inpatient rehabilitation stays, and ultimately estrangement from his wife and 2 children, with protracted periods of homelessness. The most recent episode of homelessness had occurred over the 2 years immediately before his referral to IPCC.

Ron had been drafted during the Vietnam war and served his initial period of enlistment without any medical, psychiatric, or disciplinary problems. Having completed his tour of duty in Vietnam, he reenlisted with the hope of gaining additional vocational skills and benefits. At age 22, a year into this reenlistment, he experienced an acute psychotic episode, exhibiting paranoid delusions and disorganized thought processes as well as isolative behavior, restricted affect, and avolition. Several diagnoses were considered, including schizoaffective disorder, substance-induced psychotic disorder, and major depressive disorder with psychotic features. With a diagnosis of schizophrenia, Ron was discharged with a "service-connected disability" for this medical condition. This status entitled him to both a monthly disability income and ongoing medical care from the VA.

Making the Diagnosis and Developing a Treatment Plan. After hospitalization, Ron returned home to his wife and elder child. Over the next decade, he experienced several exacerbations and hospitalizations, with disruptions to his marriage resulting in a divorce. Ron had used cocaine and alcohol intermittently during this period, but his substance use, especially cocaine use, escalated once he lost the stability and structure provided by his family. Between the ages of 30 and 45, Ron had repeated hospitalizations and drug treatment, with poor adherence to outpatient care after discharge. During this period he experienced episodes of decreased sleep, elevated mood, agitation, pressured speech, and increase in energy and goal-directed activity, as well as episodes of depressed mood, anhedonia, and decreased energy and concentration. These episodic mood symptoms appeared shortly before the reemergence of the psychotic features previously described. Consequently, the diagnosis of bipolar disorder with psychotic features was made. In addition to these symptoms, he frequently used cocaine, which caused impairment in social and relationship functioning, leading to a diagnosis of cocaine dependence. Despite his reliable disability income from the VA, poor judgment secondary to his mental illness and substance abuse contributed to many episodes of homelessness.

The turning point for Ron came 11 years ago when he was arrested for driving while intoxicated. By then he had dropped out of treatment at the VA, was not working, and stayed intermittently at his parents' home but spent most of his income and energy acquiring and using crack cocaine and alcohol. The judge ordered him into treatment in a dual-diagnosis program at a local community mental health clinic.

Initially, Ron denied that alcohol or drugs were serious problems and he resisted treatment. He focused instead solely on legal charges, unemployment, and lack of housing. The community facility recognized the need for more intensive services and recommended that he consider the IPCC program, where residential chemical dependency treatment was arranged within the VA system. Following this, Ron was eligible for referral to a halfway house and then to a supported community residence. At the residential program, Ron's neglect of long-standing health problems, including hypertension and diabetes, was recognized, and he was referred to a VA primary care clinic. Eight years ago, he finally got his own apartment.

THE PROBLEM OF HOMELESSNESS AMONG VETERANS

The extent of the problem of homelessness among the VA patient population is very large. The Northeast Program Evaluation Center (NEPEC) provides information about effectiveness of VA homeless programs. Their Web site (http://www.nepec.org/PHV/default.htm) allows access to annual reports and other information. A one-day census of VA inpatient programs (1995–2000) counted one-quarter of veterans in acute inpatient beds as homeless (U.S. Department of Veterans Affairs [VA] 2005). Ninety-seven percent of homeless veterans are male, and most are single (VA 2005). Nearly one-half of homeless veterans suffer from mental illness; greater than two-thirds of them have alcohol or drug abuse problems, and more than one-third have both psychiatric and substance abuse disorders (VA 2005).

Veterans' homelessness usually results from the same interrelated economic and personal factors that cause homelessness for other Americans.

Data from the National Vietnam Veterans Readjustment Study (NVVRS) showed that premilitary experiences had strong relationships to homelessness. Adolescent conduct disorder and childhood physical and sexual abuse revealed a greater risk for homelessness than did military experience (Rosenheck and Fontana 1994). In one survey, 31% of homeless veterans believed that military service increased their risk of homelessness, citing three aspects of their service that they believed had contributed to their homeless situation: 1) chemical misuse problems that began in the military (75%), 2) inadequate preparation for civilian employment (68%), and 3) loss of a structured lifestyle (Mares and Rosenheck 2004).

ACCESSING VA CLINICAL, HOUSING, VOCATIONAL, AND ENTITLEMENT PROGRAMS

The VA has adopted evidence-based practices such as ACT in their IPCC and other intensive case management programs and has specifically targeted homeless veterans for services. Last year, the VA operated the country's largest network of homeless assistance programs, provided health care services to about 100,000 homeless veterans, and dispersed compensation or pension benefits to more than 40,000 homeless veterans (VA 2005). Approximately 76,000 veterans receive specialized care in the VA's homeless veterans programs annually (Kasprow et al. 2005).

To develop a multidisciplinary treatment plan of the greatest benefit to the veteran, the clinician must be aware of the vast array of services offered by the VA. The following descriptions of many of these programs are adapted in whole or in part from the VA Fact Sheet "VA Programs for Homeless Veterans" (VA 2005).

General Medical and Behavioral Health Care Through the VA System

The core of general medical services at VA medical centers is the primary care clinics and their community clinics located at outlying sites beyond the main VA campuses. Utilization patterns of these services were recently reviewed (Payne et al. 2005).

Homeless veterans have significantly more chronic medical and mental health conditions, including hepatitis C, than do homeless men who are not veterans (Gish et al. 2005; O'Toole et al. 2003).

Intensive Psychiatric Community Care

IPCC was developed within the VA as a treatment delivery system for people with severe mental illness, modeled after the Program for Assertive Community Treatment (PACT) developed by Stein and Test (1980). Although this program is not exclusively for homeless individuals, a consistent finding with this model is improved housing stability (Mueser et al. 1998). IPCC provides care under four core principles: 1) high intensity of service with frequent clinician visits and low caseloads (7–15 patients per clinician); 2) flexibility and community orientation; 3) rehabilitation focus; and 4) continuity of care, with the IPCC team being the fixed point of responsibility (Rosenheck and Neale 1998). In 2000, a new initiative in mental health intensive case management (MHICM) subsumed IPCC, Intensive Community Case Management (ICCM) and other VA ACT programs (Neal et al. 2005).

The VA's Health Care for Homeless Veterans (HCHV) Program

HCHV provides extensive outreach to severely mentally ill veterans who are not currently patients at VA medical centers. Linkage is made with services such as VA clinical programs, residential treatment in community-based halfway houses, and supported housing in transitional or permanent settings; as well, treatment and rehabilitation are provided directly by program staff. Through various departments, VA staff provide physical and psychiatric exams, mental health and chemical dependency treatment referrals, and ongoing case management once the veteran is declared eligible for this service delivery system. For example, internal medicine provides general medical care including physical examinations. Psychiatry provides a multidisciplinary team that offers psychiatric assessments, chemical dependency treatment, and case management for ongoing care in the community regarding housing and entitlements. Outreach case managers for this program had approached Ron during stays at the homeless shelters and rehabilitation programs. Although he accepted some referrals for psychiatric hospitalization or chemical dependency treatment, follow-through after release remained a problem for him.

Housing Programs for Homeless Veterans

The VA sponsors a comprehensive array of housing for disabled veterans. In Ron's case, two of the programs were used on his path to recovery. After residential chemical dependency treatment, he went to a halfway house for 6 months and then to a supported community residence for a year and a half before he moved into his own apartment.

The VA's Domiciliary Care for Homeless Veterans Program (DCHV)

DCHV provides medical care and rehabilitation in a residential setting on VA Medical Center grounds to eligible veterans disabled by medical or psychiatric disorders, injury, or age. The domiciliary conducts outreach and referral; admission screening and assessment; medical and psychiatric evaluation; treatment, vocational counseling, and rehabilitation; and postdischarge community support.

Transitional Residential Facilities

Transitional residential facilities are required to assist patients until they are able to live independently. Included are halfway houses, three-quarter-way houses, cooperative apartments, crisis lodge facilities, specialized hotels, and residential care facilities. These facilities provide room and board, supervise medications, and offer assistance with activities of daily living for residents with psychiatric and developmental disabilities. Through its Homeless Providers Grant and Per Diem program, the VA makes awards to develop new homeless assistance programs. More information on applying for these grants may be obtained from the relevant page on the VA Web site (http://www1.va.gov/homeless/page.cfm?pg=3).

HUD-VA Supported Housing (VASH) Program

VASH is a joint program of the VA and the Department of Housing and Urban Development (HUD). The program provides permanent housing and ongoing treatment to mentally ill and chemically dependent homeless veterans. HUD's Section 8 Voucher Program has designated more than 1,750 vouchers worth $44.5 million for chronically mentally ill homeless veterans, and VA personnel at 34 sites provide outreach, clinical care, and case management (VA 2005).

The VA's Supported Housing Program

The VA supported housing program allows VA personnel to help homeless veterans secure long-term transitional or permanent housing. These veterans have very high rates of substance abuse and psychiatric disorders, and many have been homeless for longer than 6 months. Staff provide ongoing case management to help veterans remain in affordable housing. VA staff work with private landlords, public housing authorities, and nonprofit organizations to find housing arrangements. Veteran service organizations have also been instrumental in helping the VA establish these housing alternatives (VA 2005).

VA Vocational Programs

Vocational Rehabilitation

Homelessness is a barrier to employment because an address and phone are often required to attain employment. Shelter is required to maintain hygiene and grooming to get and hold a job, as well as regular sleep and nutrition to maintain fitness for work. Kerrigan et al. (2004) identified approximately 100 Veterans Industries work therapy programs in the Veterans Health Administration (VHA) throughout the United States. Kerrigan and colleagues studied 80 veterans who were referred to work therapy from addictions treatment programs. Besides homelessness, barriers to employment for veterans include tight job markets, drug use, age, and disability status (Kashner et al. 2002). A randomized controlled trial studied the impact of work therapy on health status among homeless, substance-dependent veterans (Kashner et al. 2002). Homeless subjects in the work therapy program, compared with nonparticipant control subjects, were more likely to initiate outpatient addictions treatment and less likely to experience substance abuse problems, report physical symptoms, and have episodes of homelessness and incarceration. In the case of veterans being discharged without marketable skills, vocational rehabilitation immediately before and/or after discharge may improve the chances of retaining housing and making a good transition to civilian life.

Compensated Work-Therapy and Transitional Residence Program

Through its Veterans Industry/Compensated Work-Therapy (VI/CWT) and Compensated Work-Therapy/Transitional Residence (CWT/TR) program, VA offers structured work opportunities and supervised therapeutic housing for at-risk and homeless veterans with physical, psychiatric, and substance abuse disorders. The VA contracts with private industry and the public sector for jobs, enabling veterans to learn new job skills and relearn successful work habits, regaining self-esteem. With a portion of their pay, veterans contribute to the maintenance and upkeep of the residence in which they live (VA 2005).

As part of this program, the VHA and the VA's National Cemetery Administration have partnered at national cemeteries to offer formerly homeless veterans in the CWT program rehabilitative work opportunities, thus providing VA cemeteries with a supplemental work force (VA 2005).

Other VA Entitlements and Outreach Programs

Veterans Benefits Assistance at VA Regional Offices

Staff members who serve as points of contact for homeless veterans provide veterans' benefits assistance. Homeless coordinators at VA regional offices provide outreach services and expedite the processing of homeless veterans' claims. The Homeless Eligibility Clarification Act allows eligible veterans without fixed addresses to receive VA checks at VA regional offices (VA 2005).

Acquired Property Sales for Homeless Providers Program

This program makes properties that the VA obtains through foreclosures on VA-insured mortgages available for sale to homeless-services providers at a discount of 20% to 50%. These properties are used to provide sheltered nights to veterans and other homeless persons (VA 2005).

Readjustment Counseling Service's Vet Centers
The Readjustment Counseling Service's Vet Centers provide outreach, counseling, supportive social services, and referrals to other VA and community programs. Every Vet Center has a homeless veterans' coordinator assigned to make sure services are tailored to local needs. The program serves more than 10,000 homeless veterans each year (VA 2005).

Stand Downs
Stand downs are one-to three-day events that provide homeless veterans a variety of services and allow both VA and community-based service providers to reach more homeless veterans. Stand downs offer a temporary refuge where homeless veterans can obtain food, shelter, clothing, and a range of community and VA assistance. In many locations, stand downs provide health screenings, referral, and access to long-term treatment, benefits counseling, ID cards, and access to other programs to meet their immediate needs. Each year, the VA participates in more than 100 stand downs coordinated by local groups (VA 2005).

VA Excess Property for Homeless Veterans Initiative
VA Excess Property provides federal excess personal property, such as clothing, footwear, sleeping bags, blankets, and other items, to homeless veterans through VA domiciliaries and other outreach activities. This initiative has been responsible for the distribution of more than $110 million in material and currently has $7 million in inventory. It also employs formerly homeless veterans to receive, warehouse, and ship these goods to VA homeless programs across the country (VA 2005).

CONCLUSION

This chapter highlights the challenges and possibilities of providing care for homeless veterans. Although military service appears to increase slightly one's risk for homelessness, especially among Vietnam, post-Vietnam, and female veterans (Mares and Rosenheck 2004), it also makes one eligible for the wide array of specialized programs for homeless veterans described. These include health care for medical and psychiatric illnesses, case management, substance abuse treatment, housing, and vocational programs. For those individuals with severe mental disorders and addictions like Ron, intensive case management through IPCC may be necessary to maintain gains in the community.

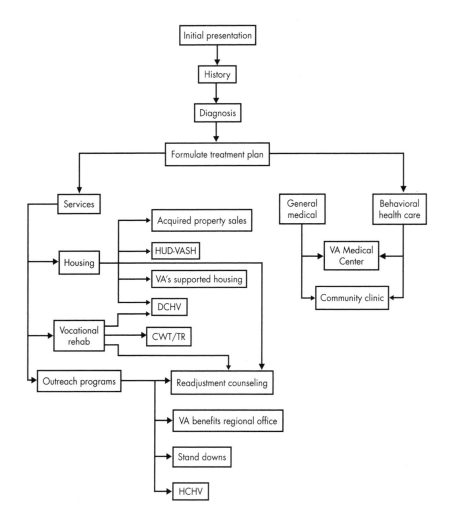

FIGURE 13–1. Flowchart: treatment and servces for homeless veterans.

CWT/TR=Compensated Work-Therapy/Transitional Residence; DCHV=Domiciliary Care for Homeless Veterans; HCHV=Health Care for Homeless Veterans; HUD-VASH=Department of Housing and Urban Development–VA-Supported Housing; VA=Department of Veterans Affairs.

Updated information on Veterans Affairs programs may be found through the VA Fact Sheets at http://www1.va.gov/opa/fact/index.htm. Updated annual reports on the Health Care for Homeless Veterans Programs are at http://www.nepec.org/PHV/default.htm under HCHV Reports.

Figure 13–1 summarizes the health care and other services available to homeless veterans. Individual VAMCs may vary in the organizational structures and services offered.

Contacting one's local VAMC Veterans Benefits Office and inquiring about services for homeless veterans will facilitate accessing care and programs for these individuals.

REFERENCES

Gish RG, Afdhal NH, Dieterich DT, et al: Management of hepatitis C virus in specialized populations: patient and treatment considerations. Clin Gastroenterol Hepatol 3:311–318, 2005

Kashner TM, Rosenheck R, Campinell AB, et al: Impact of work therapy on health status among homeless, substance-dependent veterans: a randomized controlled trial. Arch Gen Psychiatry 59:938–944, 2002

Kasprow WJ, Rosenheck R, DiLella D, et al: Health Care for Homeless Veterans Programs, Eighteenth Annual Report. April 15, 2005. West Haven, CT, Northeast Program Evaluation Center. Available at: http://www.nepec.org/PHV/default.htm. Accessed December 26, 2005.

Kerrigan AJ, Kaough JE, Wilson BL, et al: Vocational rehabilitation of participants with severe substance use disorders in a VA veterans industries program. Subst Use Misuse 39:2513–2523, 2004

Mares AS, Rosenheck RA: Perceived relationship between military service and homelessness among homeless veterans with mental illness. J Nerv Ment Dis 192:715–719, 2004

Mueser KT, Bond GR, Drake RE, et al: Model of community care for severe mental illness: a review of research on case management. Schizophr Bull 24:37–74, 1998

Neal M, Rosenheck R, Castrodonatti J, et al: Mental Health Intensive Case Management (MHICM) in the Department of Veterans Affairs: The Eighth National Performance Monitoring Report, FY 2004. West Haven, CT, Northeast Program Evaluation Center, 2005. Available at: http://www.nepec.org/MHICM/default.htm.

O'Toole TP, Conde-Martel A, Gibbon JL, et al: Health care of homeless veterans. J Gen Intern Med 18:929–933, 2003

Payne SM, Lee A, Clark JA, et al: Utilization of medical services by Veterans Health Study (VHS) respondents. J Ambul Care Manage 28:125–140, 2005

Rosenheck RA, Fontana A: A model of homelessness among male veterans of the Vietnam War generation. Am J Psychiatry 151:421–427, 1994

Rosenheck RA, Neale MS: Cost-effectiveness of intensive psychiatric community care for high users of inpatient services. Arch Gen Psychiatry 55:459–466, 1998

Stein LI, Test MA: Alternative to mental hospital treatment, I: conceptual model, treatment program, and clinical evaluation. Arch Gen Psychiatry 37:392–397, 1980

U.S. Department of Veterans Affairs [VA]: VA Fact Sheets, Programs and Issues. VA Programs for Homeless Veterans Web site, September 27, 2005. Available at: http://www1.va.gov/opa/fact/hmlssfs.html. Accessed December 9, 2005.

Chapter 14

RURAL SETTINGS

Jennifer Dempster, L.P.C.C, L.I.C.D.C.
Paulette Marie Gillig, M.D., Ph.D.

Larry, a 54-year-old man, became known to a rural community mental health and alcohol/drug agency through his sister, who was very concerned about his condition. Larry had wandered across the countryside for at least 10 years but would occasionally stay with his sister in a small town for a week or two before disappearing again for months at a time. This time Larry informed his sister he hears voices that tell him people are trying to harm him, causing him to flee. He is anxious about asking for help and is fearful that "they will lock me up and throw away the key."

UNIQUE ASPECTS OF THE SETTING: WHAT IS DIFFERENT ABOUT RURAL HOMELESSNESS?

A rural area has been defined in the U.S. Census as a nonmetropolitan area of less than 50,000 population. However, in 1990 the Census loosely subdivided rural areas into four types: 1) *rural adjacent*—contiguous to or within a metropolitan (urban) area of 50,000 population or more, 2) *rural nonadjacent*—not contiguous to a metropolitan area; 3) *urbanized rural*—with a population of 25,000 or more and not adjacent to a metropolitan area, or 4) *frontier*—fewer than six people per square mile (Post 2002; Rural Assistance Center 2006; U.S. Census Bureau 1995). In 2000, the Census defined rural areas as being "outside of urbanized areas or urbanized clusters" (U.S. Census Bureau 2002).

There are differences between homelessness in rural areas and in urban settings. Homelessness in rural areas is less visible. There are few shelters. Mentally ill homeless persons will not be found living under bridges. More

151

likely, they are living temporarily in campers or in old cars or with a succession of friends or family in overcrowded or substandard housing. "Couching it" is the term they use to describe their housing. Because homelessness is less visible in rural areas, homeless persons often are not counted in the census or other tallies. According to the Census Bureau, rural homelessness is estimated to be 7% of the overall homelessness in the United States. However, demographers estimate the actual rural rate to be around 14%. (Aron et al. 1996) In 2002, Post reported estimates describing that 9% of mentally ill homeless persons lived in rural areas, 21% in suburban areas, and 71% in central cities.

Unfortunately, despite the need for housing, less than 5% of McKinney grant funds from the U.S. Department of Housing and Urban Development go to rural communities, which often lack staff and resources necessary to compete for federal grants. The stigma of homelessness in rural settings contributes to the complexity of the problem, in that those living in campers and overcrowded housing do not identify themselves as "homeless" to the Census Bureau. Similar considerations and the complexity of the health care system often result in the homeless individual or family with mental health needs not accessing or knowing how to access appropriate referrals to community resources. Managed care systems can be a particular problem for homeless persons because families move around so much (Post 2002). Even if children are on Medicaid, they may not be able to access health care when a managed care system is in place and it is for this reason, for example, that the state of Tennessee has exempted homeless persons from Tenncare managed care rules (Post 2002).

Homeless people in rural areas who are *not* mentally ill are often white, female, married, currently working, and homeless for the first time and for a short period of time (U.S. Department of Agriculture 1996). Families, single mothers, and children make up the largest group of the rural homeless (Vissing 1996). Homeless people in rural areas tend to be older than in urban areas (over age 35), and in general there are fewer African Americans and more Native Americans. Homeless persons in rural areas are predominantly Caucasian in Appalachia and the rural areas of the Northeast and upper Midwest, African American in the Mississippi Delta. There are clusters of Native Americans in areas close to Indian reservations and of Latinos in the parts of the country that attract migrant labor (including, to some extent, Ohio) (Post 2002).

CAUSES OF RURAL HOMELESSNESS

The causes of rural homelessness are comparable to those in urban areas but in some ways different: as described by Post, in rural areas, agricultural regions that were economically dependent on declining extractive industries such as mining, timber, or fishing have lost wealth, while some economic growth areas (i.e., new industries) attracted more job seekers than could be absorbed and, as in urban areas, real estate gentrification drove up housing costs (Post 2002). This is beginning to be a problem in Larry's area, where tiny dwellings and trailers next to a small fishing lake share space with new "McMansions" and summer homes.

Other trends causing homelessness in rural areas include the lack of employment opportunities. Fitchen (1992) identified lack of transportation, restrictive land use regulations and housing codes, rising rent burdens, and insecure tenancy resulting from changes in the local real estate market (for example, the displacement of trailer park residents) as factors in rural homelessness. Bolda and colleagues (2000) have discussed the unintended consequences of more stringent building codes for poor people. For example, the cost of renovating and upgrading construction is passed on to renters. The intended beneficiaries of new "improvements" in effect may be inadvertently forced into homelessness because of increased rental costs. (Jesse Jackson said that "urban renewal" was really "urban removal," but rural areas don't have such an articulate spokesperson yet!)

As Post (2002) has illustrated, the reason that homeless shelters are virtually nonexistent in rural areas is because construction and maintenance is usually not cost-effective. Small towns with limited revenue are reluctant to encourage tax-exempt property owners and public assistance programs for fear of becoming magnets for homeless people, especially if these small towns are on heavy transportation routes (Post 2002). There are few real housing vacancies in rural areas. Metropolitan areas are more likely to have real rental units (39%) compared with nonmetropolitan areas (15%). Rural "vacancies" often are not truly vacant apartments; rather, they are for seasonal or recreational use, tourists, or migrant workers.

Rural homeless persons are more than twice as likely as urban homeless persons to be high school dropouts, are more likely to be without any health insurance, and have had the highest rates of incarcerations, with 67% having been in juvenile detention, jail or prison (Post 2002). According to Burt, homeless persons in rural areas also have higher rates of domestic violence than do homeless persons in urban settings, and substance abuse is a significant problem. Thirty-six percent of homeless rural patients report an alcohol-related problem without another psychiatric disorder. The percentage of homeless persons seen for treatment in mental health and substance abuse facilities who also report other drug problems increases as urbanization increases: the rate is 20% alcohol plus other drugs in rural settings, 35% in suburban settings, and 41% in urban settings. Slightly more than one-third of rural homeless respondents report having a mental health problem, compared with more than one-half of urban homeless persons (Burt et al. 1999). Stigmatization of mental illness and substance abuse may compromise the accuracy of these self-reports, and stigma is reportedly greater in rural than in urban areas (Wagner et al. 1995). For example, the local mental health agency had to plant landscape shrubs around the parking lot to conceal the license plates of patients' vehicles so that local residents could not cruise the highway to check to see who was receiving treatment there.

Compared with urban areas, people with severe psychiatric disorders probably constitute a smaller segment of the rural homeless, but they present special challenges (Loy 1997), as we discuss below.

DIFFERENTIAL DIAGNOSIS

Larry's situation was evaluated by an intake person at the community mental health center, then by a social work therapist and the consulting psychiatrist. He was treated as an outpatient with medication, counseling, and case management. It was learned that Larry had been actively drinking most of his life, finding that using alcohol was the only way he could tolerate the voices and "feel normal."

Larry had been brought in to the agency by his sister to be evaluated. On the basis of his auditory hallucinations, ongoing paranoid delusions, ideas of reference, and thought blocking, he was diagnosed with schizophrenia. This diagnosis was made by the consulting psychiatrist at the agency (who drives almost 70 miles one way to see patients at the agency), in consultation with the treatment team, and especially with the social work clinician who had done the intake evaluation and who interviewed Larry's sister for additional history. According to Larry's sister, Larry had been something of a loner throughout grade school and junior high school but did have a few friends. When he was about 16, he began to drink alcohol in an attempt to "calm his nerves." He dropped out of school the next year and left the family home, hitchhiking throughout the rural community and staying with relatives in different counties for short periods of time. After several breaking-and-entering episodes that involved stealing small amounts of money and food from local farmers, he was arrested. On those occasions he was intoxicated with alcohol but also appeared to be very confused and said he was hearing the voice of the devil. A crisis evaluation at the jail done by a mobile outreach worker from the rural mental health/substance abuse clinic led to a brief emergency psychiatric hospitalization in an urban community some distance from his home. He was stabilized there, but after discharge he stopped treatment, would not return for outpatient follow-up, and began to wander the community again. When he returned to his sister's place 8 months later, she brought him to the outpatient clinic for help.

After the initial intake and several follow-up home visits by an emergency case manager to his sister's home, where he was staying in the barn, he agreed to work with a dually credentialed therapist, who would help him move through the Stages of Change model (Prochaska et al. 1994) for coping with alcohol dependence and would also address treatment for schizophrenia, which he now agreed was needed because he could not stand the voices any more.

Once established as a patient, Larry was eventually stabilized on medication, became relatively abstinent (after a few relapses of alcohol use) and was linked with the ADAMH (Alcohol, Drug and Mental Health) Board housing program, where he was placed in a Transitional Rehabilitative Housing Assistance Program apartment. Later, Larry was willing to attend Intensive Outpatient Services and became sober and medication compliant, with much support from case management. He then was able to regularly attend weekly meetings of "Double Trouble," the local support group for co-occurring mental health and substance abuse disorders, with transportation provided by case management.

The housing programs that were in place to help Larry were created as part of the local homelessness coalition project, which we describe below.

SETTINGS FOR CLINICAL ENGAGEMENT

It can be difficult to engage a person with Larry's problems in treatment, and it may take even more time and patience to develop a sense of relationship when one wants to discuss the relatively fewer options available in a rural setting. In this case, even after he was established as a patient, Larry appeared and disappeared for the next 2 years, each time having a little more contact with a specific therapist at the local agency. He would talk only to this therapist because he felt he had had poor experiences previously with others at the agency. He had no other choice in agencies, this being the only provider in town that would accept him without payment.

When an individual depletes family and friend supports and the illness exacerbates further, he or she may have to make drastic decisions, especially in rural settings where there are no shelters. This may mean illegal behavior such as finding shelter in an abandoned house or barn, or looking for unlocked cars to sleep in overnight. Our agency has made mobile outreach runs to abandoned cars on the highway, in barns, and in the woods behind farms, and once we participated with all available sheriff's deputies in a two-county emergency search of all cornfields for an acutely suicidal person, homeless but with a cell phone, who had slashed her carotid artery and was unsure of her location. (She was found and airlifted to a university medical center, where she required several units of blood.) If the homeless person is also a substance abuser, the added stress of homelessness may lead to increased use, which in turn amplifies personal and public risk behaviors. Often, in rural settings, the mentally ill homeless person is met for the very first time by the mental health treatment team at the local emergency department or in jail. Compared with urban populations, rural mentally ill persons typically have higher arrest and incarceration rates by the time they receive mental health or substance abuse treatment. Sixty-seven percent of rural homeless persons have been in juvenile detention, jail, or prison (Post 2002). Sometimes this incarceration is seen as a mission of mercy by the sheriff's deputy when it is bitter cold and there are no other options. Creative and sometimes rather whimsical "charges" are filed to give the homeless person a cot in the jail over-night, including our perennial favorite, "leaning with intent to fall."

DEVELOPING COMMUNITY TEAMWORK STRATEGIES

Larger cities that have had to be responsible for shelter services to areas be-yond their municipal borders also have rural persons utilizing their services (i.e., "taking up beds"). This has motivated some urban housing programs to work with the rural settings to better manage resources, developing collabo-rations instead of boundaries. Examples of collaborations include the SKY-CAP program in Hazard, Kentucky (a rural, nonadjacent area), where case management works with sheltered and unsheltered homeless people in neigh-boring counties in which much of the topography is vertical. As Post (2002) describes:

> Three organizations coordinate a voluntary network of more than 80 agencies and service providers through a management information system that tracks social service, housing, and clinical and environmental factors that affect the health of people who are homeless and at risk of homelessness. (p. 22)

Another HUD-funded approach to rural homelessness has been the Mul-tiservice Center. The Homeless HealthCare program in Burlington, Ver-mont, works with the one-third of the homeless population who are from rural areas throughout the state (rural adjacent and rural nonadjacent). Post (2002) describes this model:

> All mental health, substance abuse, case management, and primary care ser-vices are coordinated at a single point of access. A pro bono network of pri-vate practitioners provides mental health services. (p. 22)

The "hub and spoke model" described by Post (2002) is used in Mon-tana, an entirely rural state with large frontier areas (rural frontier):

> The Yellowstone City-County Health Department's Homeless Healthcare project in Billings and its sub-grantees in Helena, Butte and Missoula have a hub and spoke model that serves homeless people who migrate to these cities from outlying areas, using a mobile van to reach out to unsheltered persons in remote areas. All towns with homeless health care projects have specialists within their provider network. These overlap with the responsibilities of com-munity health centers, health departments, homeless health care, and Indian

and migrant health services. This fosters a high degree of collaboration and service integration. (pp. 22–23)

The U.S. Department of Housing and Urban Development (2004) has encouraged all communities to develop a comprehensive, integrated system of care to reduce homelessness called the Continuum of Care. The system is developed through collaboration with a broad cross-section of the community and is based on a thorough assessment of homeless needs and resources. When the Continuum of Care can be established, the community can then proactively make decisions about specific problems and needs and can address them collectively, instead of single agencies' having to deal with a crisis alone. This process also leads to a greater buy-in of the community as a whole. Particularly in rural communities, unless collaboration is developed, homelessness cannot be managed and remains a day-to-day crisis.

RURAL HOMELESSNESS COALITIONS

In Ohio, both Logan and Champaign counties developed rural coalitions, which, taken together, became their Continuum of Care program. The local community leaders, including the newspaper publishers and police, were eager to get involved to solve the homelessness problem in their community. The director of the homelessness program was and is a clinically licensed counselor and also a clergyman, originally working for the community mental health /alcohol and drug agency as a case management supervisor. The director contracted with the ADAMH Board through an existing housing program to provide some housing units. After some time it became evident the rural standalone program could not address the problem alone. At this point, a rural-urban coalition was formed with a homelessness agency in Dayton, Ohio. Dayton is an urban area in relatively close proximity to many rural communities, including Logan and Champaign counties.

One of the activities having the most impact locally was the Point in Time study described below.

THE POINT IN TIME STUDY: SMALL NUMBERS, BIG IMPACT

This study was a one-day evaluation of homelessness in the rural community. The list of homeless persons thus evaluated was then separated into categories such as mental illness, substance abuse, and medical conditions. On January 27, 2005, Champaign County, with an estimated population of 39,645 (Ohio Department of Development 2005), had 154 homeless persons, and

Logan County, with an estimated population of 46,616 (Ohio Department of Development 2005) had 197. The total number in both counties with mental illness and/or substance abuse was 78. This was surprising, because the percentage of mentally ill persons among the homeless population in Logan County was substantially higher than average, according to the 2000 U.S. Census report (U.S. Census Bureau 2002). Also, in terms of expected overall proportion of homeless persons to the total local population in any Ohio county (rural or urban), both counties were above average. In Ohio, the expected point-in-time population percentage of homeless persons is approximately 0.00245% of a country's population on any given night (Coalition on Homelessness and Housing in Ohio [COHHIO] 2001). Calculating these estimates, we found that Champaign County had a 58% higher homeless rate and Logan County had a 78% higher homeless rate than the national average.

Through this survey, the team also was able to determine what areas needed to be the focus of a strategic plan for their rural setting. The urban center in Dayton helped the rural coalition to write a successful HUD grant, which enabled the rural community to develop a significant number of housing opportunities that would not have been available without the help of the urban partnership. It was to the advantage of the urban community to help the rural area, because increased rural housing capacity relieves pressure on urban shelter beds.

ACCESS TO ENTITLEMENTS IN RURAL SETTINGS: DEVELOPING CREATIVE HOUSING OPTIONS

To create housing opportunities, one successful option in rural areas has been to develop contracts with local property owners in which an agency pays a monthly rate for sleeping rooms used as temporary housing until other arrangements are made. This gives the individual and the agency flexibility to better prepare the person for more adequate housing. When used as a hospital discharge option, this also considerably reduces cost. Financial support for this placement may be developed through local board funding, through charitable grants, or through coalitions where area agencies, faith-based organizations, and others support the effort with smaller financial contributions.

In some rural localities, including this one, the faith-based community can be a strong resource when mobilized, working cooperatively to temporarily house people for brief periods, whether in members' homes or from money set aside to help those in need, sometimes in a low-cost hotel or motel. As soon as the problem was identified, these sorts of initiatives began.

TRANSITION TO PERMANENT HOUSING

Larry maintained sobriety, after a few relapses, and was able to stay in transitional housing. He continued to be stable in his mental health symptoms and had applied for Supplemental Security Income (SSI) and Metropolitan housing. While waiting for SSI, Larry was encouraged to think about a move toward permanent housing and greater independence as required by the policies of the housing program. He saw this as a threat to his now-valued new home and disappeared from treatment for 2 weeks. When he finally contacted his therapist, he stated, "I knew you were gonna help me out just long enough to jerk the rug from underneath of me. I would have been better off living on the streets." The therapist was able to help Larry understand the nature of temporary housing and explained that he had up to 18 months to attain permanent housing and that his treatment team would work with him to attain this. Larry came back grudgingly at first, but he was able to stay in transitional housing until he received SSI and could move into permanent housing with his Section 8 housing voucher.

Transitioning to permanent housing can present greater issues than attaining temporary placement. For homeless persons, giving up ownership of anything can be a major challenge in that any possession is highly valued, as the following vignette illustrates:

Don had struggled for some time to get a job now that he had found some temporary housing with his ex-girlfriend. Finally he was able to get a job at a local factory, making more money than he had ever made before. The night before his first day of work, he and his ex-girlfriend got into a fight and she threatened to throw all his possessions out onto the street. He decided not to go to work for fear of her following through on her threats. When the therapist questioned whether what he had was so valuable that it could not be taken with him to work or replaced, he said, "It's just my things, you know, clothes and stuff." When the therapist then asked if it was worth it, Don said, "I could have bought everything I had at her house with my first paycheck, but I just could not deal with losing all that I had right then."

The idea of moving from something that is known, stable, and secure to what others define as "permanent" can often be threatening and anxiety-provoking, which can lead to mistrust. Although transitional housing may last only up to 24 months, for those who have been homeless, it feels like permanency. It is therefore important that the individual understand how the "transitional" process works. This may mean explaining the process repeatedly in different ways, having the person repeat it back as he or she interprets it. Developing a written plan can also be helpful to a person moving through the process. Fear of change and of the unknown can challenge anyone's ability to make life-improving decisions; this is no different for homeless individuals. Our agency has struggled with the idea of enforcing the rules about temporary housing, and in the past case managers have sometimes been reluctant to bring up the subject with homeless persons of their needing to move to another place. However, because of funding rules there is little choice, so with homeless persons it is very important to be sure they understand the housing rules up front so that they do not become too attached to the temporary place and despondent when they must move again.

Figure 14–1 illustrates access to rural community housing services in two Ohio counties. Typically, in rural settings, those in need of housing are evaluated by mental health agencies if the person is seen to be "at risk" or in crisis. Once entered into the system, agencies collaborate to move the individual or family through this process to attain housing as quickly as possible.

OBSTACLES IN WORKING WITH HOMELESS MENTALLY ILL PERSONS IN A RURAL MENTAL HEALTH SETTING

Helen was awarded disability because of severe depression and medical conditions. She had been a beautician for many years and was proud of her hard work in this career. Since her disability she has attempted work, but because of the combination of ruptured discs and depression, she has been unable to meet the expectations of her employers, often becoming more depressed and being rehospitalized for psychiatric reasons. She qualifies for $18 per month in food stamps, and although she jokes about the amount, she is thankful. Helen has been paying more than 70% of her check for rent in a sleeping room. The rest of her income pays utilities, food, and transportation costs. Often she has been unable to meet all of her expenses, and she had become dependent on the high-interest cash-advance payday loan stores before her Supplemental Security Income check was available each month. She had been on the Metropolitan housing waiting list for 2 years and was recently told she would be receiving a Section 8 voucher. The next month, she was informed that her voucher had been retracted because housing funds were exhausted. She would receive her voucher again when funding was restored.

She was afraid to be around the others living in her current housing complex, who would smoke marijuana at the kitchen table, steal her food, and leave a mess, which often she cleaned up. Her only hope was that she would be able to get a place of her own. Feeling hopeless and helpless, Helen became suicidal and was hospitalized again. Her sleeping room was rented to someone else during her hospitalization, and she was again homeless.

Obstacles to appropriate treatment and rehabilitation in a rural setting include lack of resources and a misunderstanding of services by agencies, such as the welfare department, that refer homeless people. Expectation about

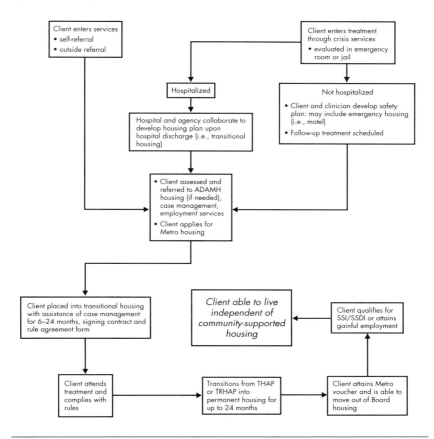

FIGURE 14–1. Flowchart: accessing rural community ADAMH Board housing services in Logan and Champaign counties, Ohio.

ADAMH=Alcohol, Drug and Mental Health; SSI=Supplemental Security Income; SSDI=Social Security Disability Insurance; THAP=Transitional Housing Assistance Program; TRHAP=Transitional and Rehabilitative Housing Assistance Program.

housing availability is an example. A homeless person with mental illness and/or alcohol and drug issues may come into the community mental health treatment facility expecting to access housing very rapidly, only to find waiting lists or lack of housing. The frustrated individual knows that his or her basic need for housing is unmet and is understandably resentful, and the provider staff may react counter-responsively and think the homeless person is "looking for a free ride" for housing without interest in treatment.

To further illuminate rural housing issues, it is useful to understand that although the cost of rent is less than in urban areas, average income is lower, equalizing differences. In rural settings, 23% of poor-homeowner households and 27% of poor-renter households occupy inadequate housing, compared with 17% and 22% in urban areas (Aron and Fitchen 1996). In our setting in Ohio, a poor person renting a typical two-bedroom unit in Logan County or Champaign County pays $536 a month. To live above the poverty line and maintain such housing, this person would have to work 81 hours per week at minimum wage, if he or she could find a job.

Moreover, those who live under the poverty line are not far from meeting definitions of homelessness. Currently the federal poverty guideline for 100% below the poverty line for an individual is $798 per month, which is $4.60 an hour. Minimum wage is currently $5.15 an hour (http://www.dol.gov/compliance/laws/comp-flsa.htm). Supplemental Security Income (SSI) and Social Security Disability Insurance (SSDI) theoretically permit a person to be "taken care of," although the average monthly income for a person on SSI is less than $600. In 2000, people in Ohio with disabilities who had SSI benefits received an average of $512 per month and needed to pay an average of 86.1% of their monthly SSI benefit to rent a 1-bedroom apartment (O'Hara and Miller 2001).

CONCLUSION

It is our hope that this chapter will contribute to a better understanding of the characteristics of rural homelessness associated with mental illness and/or substance abuse. In rural communities, homelessness of this type can be an unseen but deeply felt problem (Wagenfeld 2000). Successful programs in Ohio, Kentucky, and Montana have been built on a foundation of community collaboration and outreach. In contrast, programs often fail when the community does not support the cause and is not involved in the planning stages. Homeless persons who feel rejected upon entrance to any rural agency or community program will believe that all programs will reject them and will not pursue further support that is actually available to them. As a result, the community will then have to deal with the various crises related to the fact that homeless mentally ill persons in their area are not receiving services. A community coalition that is built on collaboration and outreach can not only reduce homelessness, but also reduce the associated community-level crises and free up resources (including the police) to help with other community needs.

REFERENCES

Aron LY, Fitchen JM: Rural homelessness: a synopsis, in Homelessness in America. Edited by Baumohl J. London, Oryx Press, 1996, pp 81–85

Bolda W, Salley S, Keith R, et al: Creating affordable rural housing with services: options and strategies. Research and Policy Brief. working paper #19, Maine Rural Health Research Center–Institute for Health Policy. Portland, University of Southern Maine, 2000

Burt MR, Laudan L, Douglas T, et al: Homelessness: programs and the people they serve: summary report. Findings of the National Survey of Homeless Assistance Providers and Clients. Washington, DC, Urban Institute, 1999

Coalition on Homelessness and Housing in Ohio (COHHIO): How Many Ohioans Experience Homelessness? 2001. Available at: http://www.cohhio.org/resources/howmanyhomeless-html.

Fitchen JM: On the edge of homelessness: rural poverty and housing insecurity. Rural Sociology 57:173–193, 1992

Loy M: Rural veterans: outreach and treatment. Vet Center Rural Veterans Working Group 18(2):2–6, 1997

O'Hara A, Miller E: Priced Out in 2000: The Crisis Continues. Technical Assistance Collaborative, Inc., and Consortium for Citizens With Disabilities Task Force, 2001. Available at: http://www.c-c-d.org/POin2000.html.

Ohio Department of Development: 2005 Ohio County Profiles. Research and Data Office of Strategic Research. Available at: http://www.odod.state.oh.us/research.

Post P: Hard to Reach: Rural Homelessness and Health Care. Nashville, TN, National Health Care for the Homeless Council (P.O. Box 60427, Nashville, TN 37206), 2002

Prochaska JO, Norcross JC, DiClemente CC: Changing for Good. New York, William Morrow, 1994

Rural Assistance Center: What Is Rural? 2006. Available at: http://www.raconline.org/info-guides/ruraldef.

U.S. Census Bureau: Urban and Rural Definitions. 1995. Available at: http://www.census.gov/population/censusdata/urdef.txt.

U.S. Census Bureau: Urban Area Criteria for Census 2000. 2002. Available at: http://www.census.gov/geo/www/ua/uafedreg031502.txt.

U.S. Department of Agriculture, Rural Economic and Community Development: Rural America: Focusing on the Needs of the Rural Homeless. Washington, DC, U.S. Department of Agriculture, 1996

U.S. Department of Housing and Urban Development: Continuum of Care Materials. Community Planning and Development Web page, 2004. Available at: http://www.hud.gov/offices/cpd/homeless/library/coc/index.cfm.

Vissing YM: Out of Sight, Out of Mind: Homeless Children and Families in Small-town America. Lexington, University Press of Kentucky, 1996

Wagenfeld M: Delivering mental health services to persistently and seriously mentally ill in frontier areas. J Rural Health 16:91–96, 2000

Wagner JD, Menke EM, Ciccone JK: What is known about the health of rural homeless families? Public Health Nurs 12:400–408, 1995

AFTERWORD

It has been, as Dr. Lamb points out in the Foreword, over 20 years since the formation of the first American Psychiatric Association Task Force and the publication of *The Homeless Mentally Ill*. At the time, I was working in Emergency Department at San Francisco General Hospital and beginning to organize San Francisco's Health Care for the Homeless program. I think a few of us remember how naïve we were at that time, and how little information was available to assist those providing services for people with severe and persistent mental illnesses and no place to live. Eighteen American cities received funding from the Robert Wood Johnson foundation to set up health care for the homeless services then; only San Francisco had included a provision for providing mental health care in addition to physical health and social work services. Those of us providing street outreach or crisis intervention were, quite literally, engaged in continuous "on-the-job training." There were no textbooks, few articles, and, in fact, only a very small peer group to whom we could turn for information and advice. The APA Task Force Report served as the first bible of service providers to the mentally ill homeless population. We were all "generalists" then, there being little information, few established clinical techniques, and few service options available.

In reading this volume, I find myself struck with two conflicting thoughts and emotions: pride in how much we've learned, and concern about all that still needs to be done. Drs. Gillig and McQuistion have assembled an impressive array of experienced experts in this textbook, many of them the national leaders in their content areas. Many have spent more than a decade providing services to homeless men and women. Each has written about his or her work and has provided major contributions to the literature on clinical care for this population. Never before, however, has so much collective wisdom and experience been provided in one volume. The editors have done us, and the field, proud.

Although chapters are arranged primarily by service site, each includes clinical pearls applicable far beyond any one type of facility. Critical themes of individualization, continuity of care, the building of interpersonal trust, and an emphasis on rehabilitation and recovery build throughout the volume.

Recognition of the contributions of others, and of the growing base of clinical and experimental evidence to inform our practice, provides a unique opportunity for today's, and tomorrow's, practitioners. Now we are no longer wayfarers whistling in the dark, individually struggling to discover the best way to take care of those we're charged with treating. Rather, what emerges is a sense of clinicians in this field being part of a larger effort, fueled by caring and compassion, but guided by accumulated experience and knowledge.

Beyond the sheer comprehensiveness of this work, what stands out for me is the use of clinical flowcharts. Certainly, "evidenced-based practice" is the buzzword of our time. However, all too often, what this has come to mean is the application of small quanta of research data to individual medication, or placement, or "type of therapy" decisions. Treatment algorithms are the rage in psychopharmacology, but rarely has the same approach been targeted for overall clinical decision making, and never before to work with homeless mentally ill individuals. I found myself, after each chapter, picking cases from my own experience, walking them through the flowchart, comparing my procedures, and decisions, with the authors'. If the true value of a text is not only the questions it answers, but the extent to which it fosters further growth in those who read it, these authors have succeeded.

Reading this work, however, was not entirely an enjoyable or satisfying experience. It is commonly acknowledged, and frequently expressed among those working with the most disenfranchised and disaffiliated populations, that one cannot do this work without becoming, somehow, politicized. Having populations go untreated because of our lack of knowledge, or technical shortcomings, or limitations to our clinical skills, is a reality to which every clinician must adjust. Working in the streets and shelters of San Francisco in the 1980s, one could not avoid experiencing the death of many clients. AIDS was only recently named, its etiology was not known, and such interventions as one could offer were palliative at best. As a clinician, one could rage, or feel impotent, but there simply were no treatments available. Now, facing the reality of huge population centers in other parts of the world going without HIV treatment despite the availability of effective interventions evokes a far different response. Now, HIV is no longer a condition whose fatality is a function of our ignorance. Now, deaths reflect our lack of will.

Similarly, it is clear that we now do know how to tackle many of the problems faced by those who are mentally ill and homeless. We have learned the value of case management, of supported housing, of building individual relationships that foster treatment adherence and residential stability. We know how to help clients learn new skills, gain symptom relief, enter rehabilitation and participate in their own recovery. This is no longer a field of uncharted terrain. Now, we fail because we won't, not because we can't, address these issues.

Much is written about the societal stigmatization of the seriously mentally ill. Far less a focus of attention in our professional literature is the marginalization of the impoverished. Alas, we know the solution to homelessness. Housing. Undomiciled mentally ill individuals, when provided a safe and affordable place to live, remain mentally ill. We know how to work with mentally ill individuals, to engage, rehabilitate, treat them. Addressing poverty remains outside of our expertise as mental health professionals. It cannot, however, remain peripheral to our commitment as citizens, as caretakers, and as better-informed members of our communities. Dr. Lamb, in his Foreword, writes: "It is my hope that the availability of this new guide to clinical care will greatly increase society's efforts to take meaningful action to help persons with severe mental illness who are homeless." It is my hope that it will serve to focus, and strengthen, our efforts, as clinicians and responsible members of that society, to move beyond our individual interventions, and bring our experience as public health practitioners to foster that change.

Stephen M. Goldfinger, M.D.

REFERENCES

Lamb HR (ed): The Homeless Mentally Ill: A Task Force Report of the American Psychiatric Association. Washington, DC, American Psychiatric Association, 1984

Lamb HR: Foreword, in Clinical Guide to the Treatment of the Mentally Ill Homeless Person. Edited by Gillig PM, McQuistion HL. Washington, DC, American Psychiatric Publishing, 2006, pp xxiii–xxiv

INDEX

*Page numbers printed in **boldface** type refer to tables or figures.*